COVID 19 ECHOES

FROM MY JOURNAL

BOOK I

BELLE MAYNARD CURD

Printed in the United States of America.

Library of Congress Control Number: 2022939649

ISBN	Paperback	978-1-68536-607-0
	Hardback	978-1-68536-608-7
	eBook	978-1-68536-609-4

Westwood Books Publishing LLC
Atlanta Financial Center
3343 Peachtree Rd NE Ste 145-725
Atlanta, GA 30326

www.westwoodbookspublishing.com

CONTENTS

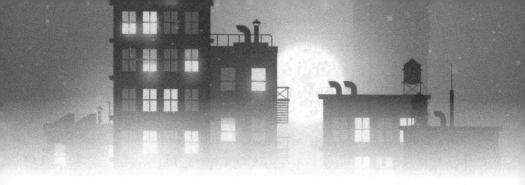

Time goes by fast. Soon (I hope) COVID-19 will pass into history. People will tell their children about the modern pandemic that traversed the world, whereby millions died, more than in all the recent wars. It will be compared to the Spanish flu of 1914 and 1915. Stories will compare the same experiences and the differences and what we learned from them.

A handful of people will know stories of child diseases before inoculations, like scarlet fever, measles, mumps, chicken pox, and more recently, SARS and the flu of 1954.

As a director of a writing group in Tsawwassen in Delta British Columbia, Canada, I always encouraged the members to write their life history. Although the public library where the meetings were held has been closed to the public, I hope they have continued to write their experiences during COVID-19 for themselves and posterity. Everyone will have a different story regarding their experiences beginning in the year 2019—hence the name. One thing that we'll agree on is being shocked and perplexed when we realized what was happening. However, in each of our compositions, there will be an accounting, either large or small of COVID-19—something that no one would like to go through again.

In order to fully understand my account, I'd like you to know a little about my background, for without it, my experience could have been quite different. I might even throw in a bit about my classmates although I haven't seen any of the members since this all started. I can't mention any notable or notorious characters whose names have bandied around in these early days of COVID. The truth is, everyone has been affected.

There is no better time to start than January 1, 2020. Now, 2020 usually carries a positive connotation. They say, "He or she has 20-20 vision," which means they have great eyesight. When it comes to COVID-19, though, it's quite the opposite. We didn't see this coming at all.

For instance, my relatives across the line in the United States are generally great about keeping in touch via email, Facebook, slow-mail, or crow-mail in their neck of the woods. Well, one of my nieces, who we'll call Ivy, wrote to the rest of us saying she was feeling ill with the flu and that it seemed like everybody was catching the flu and a friend was in the hospital there in Washington State. It didn't seem too unusual.

In hindsight, I recall that Washington State was the first to realize something wasn't just right. With SeaTac airport very busy bringing people in and out from many countries around the world they were probably the first to get hit by COVID.

My cousin Barbara in Coquitlam, British Columbia, had been in the hospital not long before—in 2019. She turned ninety-three years old last August and doesn't believe in flu shots. I gasped when she told me, but she says they make her sick. It seems she always gets better but has been in the hospital more than I like to hear.

My friend in Richmond, British Columbia, was suffering from a terrible cough that wouldn't go away although she had been to the doctor several times. She coughed and coughed. She helps the local theatre where local actors put on performances and she shows the audience to their seats. Her condition was disconcerting.

Then, tragedy appeared in my own life. My oldest son, who lives two hours east of Vancouver was been hit by a hit-and-run truck as he stepped off the curb on the main street of Mission, B.C. on his way home at 8:30 at night. He was left for dead in the middle of the road until some good Samaritans who had seen the accident hurried to his aid, bundled him up, and dialled 911. He was air-lifted to the hospital in New Westminster, clinging to life with multiple broken bones and a badly-damaged brain.

A friend from church and his young son were also hurt in a car accident in about the same vicinity and also air-lifted out, one to the same hospital as my son. Terrible as it was, COVID-19 wasn't known of at that time—at least not in Canada. It was just an ordinary weekend when father and son went to a camp meeting for young men and their fathers. No one could imagine what lay ahead.

By some miracle, my son's accident was recorded on film, not on someone's cell phone as sometimes happens on television but from a camera that was above the street on a building. The police have the make and year of the truck but because of the angle, not the license plate. My daughter spent days trying to find the driver to no avail. It was so important that he turn himself in, as my son had recently moved back to the Lower Mainland from Japan and it was too early to have his medical papers in order. Miraculously, he survived but suffered considerable brain injuries.

We still hadn't heard the word *COVID* and had no clue as we drove up to the hospital along Highway 7 driven by my second son and his wife, who were visiting from Alberta. It had been years since I was in that hospital, and many changes had been made, though much remained the same. It was like a strange city with underground parking and walkways down to the Sky Train, huge corridors and elevators everywhere. The regulation sanitary station was at every entrance. We were sure to sterilize our hands before going into the ward. We were prepared for anything but were surprised by how great he looked under the circumstances. We were happy to think that he might be able to pull through, although both legs seemed to be broken. The place was so quiet. Everyone seemed to be resting. Nurses were shuffling towards the windows. Anyone who has been in that hospital will know what I mean by the windows. They are, indeed, special.

Going home though, we travelled along 4th Ave. People on the street seemed to be wearing masks like the Orientals wore when they had a cough. *Strange*, I thought. Sure enough, it was only days before word crept in across CBC Radio and CHEK Television in Victoria about this strange disease that no one knew much about. That Sunday, my friend Susi, who took me to church in her car, said that it had come from China—from animals, maybe pigs or a market in some city I'd never heard of. No one seemed immune to it; not even the doctors seemed immune to it. They thought, at first, it would be like ordinary flu and that there wouldn't be many casualties. However, it spread without knowing any boundaries. Susi's brother, who was working in the hospital, was found contagious. He was very sick and was put in quarantine in China. No one could go near him. It was likened to the Black Death in Europe long ago when millions of people perished. I remember seeing the place where they were buried in a huge strip of land near Buckingham Palace where no one was allowed to walk because it was sacred ground. I think it was called Green Park, a strange name for a place filled with so much death. I hoped this story does not end thusly.

In the future, I may make a chart showing the dates and places for plagues across the earth with information about each plague. It should be interesting, but as far as I know, my ancestors wouldn't have a connection to them. Therefore, this is my story. I can't connect my ancestors to the Black Death. I just don't know when or how.

Skip ahead to my grandma, Jessie, and grandpa, Alexander Smith, who was a dairy farmer in the western United States. They weren't really my grandparents, but they raised my Aunt Minnie (born in 1891) and my mother, Mabel Belle (whom I have no birth record of). The Smiths travelled around the frontier from Wisconsin to Minnesota to Saskatchewan and everywhere between.

Their census papers are available in those different places, but they ended back in Mora, Minnesota. Where my mother came from, I do not know, and if she knew, she never told us. One thing the Smiths told her was that she had had diphtheria and survived. That's why I mentioned them at all in the COVID context. Did your mother ever recite the ditty, "Now I lay me down to sleep; pray the Lord my soul to keep. If I die before I awake, bless me, Lord, my soul to take."

That's how fragile life was not so long ago. We have so much to be thankful for.

Grandpa and Grandma Smith moved to Riverhurst, Saskatchewan, in 1912—just in time for the Regina Cyclone from his farm by Lake Superior, Minnesota, where a zoo now stands. They left because the government required all farmers to have their cow milk pasteurized in the United States.

Now, this was in the interest of better health, but many farmers were against pasteurization, and he was one of them. He thought he was right, and that goes down a generation or more, so I remember when I was young and inoculations came into common use that my mother wouldn't allow my sister or me to get the inoculations. The school nurse was there to inoculate all of us, but unlike now, they wouldn't force anyone to have them. I'm sure you recognize the similarity today. Some people won't take the COVID shot either. Pity!

As a result of us not having our inoculations, my sister Dot and I pretty well had every childhood disease—whooping cough, measles, mumps. We didn't have scarlet fever by some twist of fate, but those who did had to be quarantined for quite a spell. In fact, the whole family was quarantined. The father of the house who was the wage earner had to leave the family and stay away until the last child in the family was out of quarantine. I believe my brother Clarence had to go into the Regina General Hospital. Aggie was left to look after the rest of the children. Measles sometimes caused blindness. Chicken pox also caused shingles in later life. I got my first inoculation when I was nineteen years old and about to marry Bill Hogg, who was in the Navy. They never fooled around or asked permission when it came to shots. My older sisters who lived with their dad, Chester, didn't receive shots, and when Helen was ninety years old, she got shingles. It's not a happy thing to happen as anyone will tell you who has had them. My sister-in-law, Madeleine, also got shingles about the same time, I believe. Apparently, the germ stays in your body all your life.

When I heard about the damage it could do, I hurried to the pharmacy, but inoculations weren't available at that time. They were waiting for the fluid to come in. I waited and waited. That would have been around 1979. I wasn't willing to wait any longer, so when we went down south that winter, I went to a pharmacist there in California and got the protection I wanted. I remember it was expensive, but I never regretted it.

If you see a resemblance to COVID, I understand. Many people say they're not going to take the shot. I hope reading this book will make a difference. However, I wonder, as only a 37percent of the population had had their flu shot last year in 2019, and it was free. This chapter in the book has been written in 2020.

I sometimes think that this pandemic might last even longer than some people figure. I for one thought that once we got the serum, we would be free. Others make an educated guess that it will take much longer to get it distributed, and my uneducated guess that more than 40 percent will refuse the serum once it is offered . . . if history is any indication. I hope I'm wrong for everyone's sake.

Although it wasn't in our upbringing, once I had children, medically they were partially under the care of the Navy medics, as was my Navy husband. I just fell in line and was happy I had. We travelled a lot and were often required to take shots before we left. In Halifax, I remember the children had measles, so it wasn't tightly administered even under the Queen's Navy in Slackerfax, as they called Halifax in those days. Many families moved in and out of Halifax, and a few might have gotten missed in the shuffle. We lived in an old log cabin on Melville Cove Road, and there were two very sick toddlers who were blinded by the light until they got well. When they got to scrapping, I knew they would get better, and soon they were running around as usual. The measles was over.

I was so happy but I would have been happier if they'd had their inoculations. They could have died or been blinded then or in later life. Measles is more dangerous than it was once believed to be.

Doctor Bonnie Henry, our medical officer (I'm not sure of her title), and Adrian Dix, our public health officer and member of Parliament for British Columbia, got together with the British Columbia Centre for Disease Control, working through details about the public needing to know as much information about this pandemic that was flooding the city, the province, and of course, Canada on the whole—not to mention our neighbour south of us, the United States, and Britain, France, and Italy in particular. How were they to protect themselves from getting COVID? What is the cure? If they get it, is there some medicine we can take? How can we not get it?

Do all these pieces fall into place? Will your COVID story be different? I'm sure it will. The best thing the government has done (as far as I'm concerned) was lowering the interest rates the banks charge. House sales have been surging forward in the last few months. That must help a lot of buyers and sellers. Actually, there is a shortage of housing. It may not help house construction, as the cost of lumber in Canada has increased exponentially, so it's much more expensive to buy a lot and build a new home than it was a year ago. Maybe rates will go down a little further. I'll be surprised if they do. Some institutions have already put in operation increases as soon as the pandemic is over, and every year after that. In the United States, you can get a mortgage for thirty years, but in Canada, the rate can only be assured for five years or less.

Renters, too, have been helped, I believe. I have found that owners cannot increase the rent for their tenants. However, I've noticed that it hasn't hindered apartment managers from increasing rates to owners. I don't believe municipal rates have increased, which is something else to be thankful for. It was never imagined that COVID could go on for this long. As many restaurants were closing, many more people were without work. The government often encouraged people to go out and spend, on one hand, to help keep the economy running and on the other hand, not to go anywhere near other people, except those from immediate families and those like medical helpers—necessary workers who had no choice but to leave their homes. Many people who could manage it, were working from their homes. Schools were closed. Students took their classes on the Internet as far as possible. Play schools for the little ones and Day Cares were regulated. The streets were empty of cars. Buses ran almost empty. The number of stops was decreased. We were all encouraged to stay two metres away from each other and not to visit families given certain numbers.

Care Homes for the elderly were the hardest hit.

I continued to play a little game and tried to live a financial life like I had lived while in university. I had started to cut back some about a year before, as I was getting deeper in debt and my line of credit at the local bank was going up and up. I hadn't gone into any stores save the grocery store and the odd trip to a dollar store with the excuse that I didn't drink, I didn't smoke, and I was benefitting from their endless selection of cheap goods. I didn't go there very often but when I did, I felt I was saving a lot of money.

I needed a new walker, as the wheels had gone on my one hand-me-down and the other one had also seen better days. I dreamed about the stores I would visit when this was all over.

I kept doing little things to spend as little as possible as if we are even poorer than we were. I washed my clothes in cold water, which I learned from my daughter, and dried them outside on a rack to save electricity and cut the furnace back to a reasonable temperature. I even tried to save water use. That was rather silly, but Vancouver has to pay for the water we used, as it came off the mountains in North Vancouver. We're probably one of the luckiest cities in the world. I tried to put the recyclables in the right bin and all the green materials in the green container. Not wasting food, especially fruit and vegetables was difficult, I'll admit. All scrap paper had its own container.

A lot of people never mail any letters these days. Email sure helps, as no stamp is needed. I still enjoy letters and cards. I have trouble remembering everyone's birthday, COVID or no COVID. I must repent.

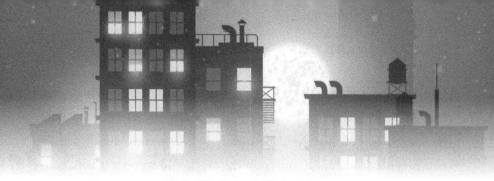

ELECTIONS

The United States election was coming up—just two weeks away. I believed it would be quite a mess but what happens in the States definitely affects Canada, along with the rest of the world (especially the Mexicans trying to get into the US). President Donald Trump bragged about paying so little income tax. In 1997, I was in the top 1 percent in paying income tax as I had sold some properties so you can say I was very jealous of him. I'll admit that, in a sense, I didn't feel good about it, but I felt good about being that little person who rose from the daughter whose mother cleaned floors for a living and told me her reason for raising me was to finish school and look after her. I did have the privilege of sharing the vestibule of the Bellagio in Las Vegas and to see Donald I think he was talking to his cohorts about his real estate empire and to be a witness to the building of his big hotel in Waikiki between the hotel I was in and my view of the grand Pacific . . . I can't say I liked him after that. The things he did prior to the election didn't improve my impression of him either.

In the meantime, COVID and my friend's perpetual cough took precedent as I swung by her house in Richmond, not far from my house, and noticed she had a terrible cough and complications. Not much later, I had the same symptoms. Could it be that COVID monster threatening our lives? Eventually, I thought it might be from the construction going on across the lane from my backyard, day in and day out. The table on the back porch was always filthy—dirty every time I washed it. The car parked out back was a disgrace to drive down the road it was so dirty and had been found to have a nail piercing the tire with only 22,000 miles on the clock. No wonder it kept going flat. Add to this fact that California, Oregon, and Washington were suffering from the greatest fires in history, so there was black smoke in the air even though we were far north of those states. Miraculously, I hadn't heard of anyone losing their lives—a miracle in itself—but thousands of homes were burned to the ground. Everyone knew enough to move out when warned to do so.

Families had escaped in their vehicles, often with whatever they could salvage in a matter of moments. Men there to fight the fire weren't so fortunate. They often received lung damage when fighting the flames. We realized the damage a thousand miles away on television and even when the sky darkened day after day We knew the sun was up there but only faint fiery orange shadow where the sun used to be no more than a hint. The elderly were warned not to leave the house. Deaths multiplied in care homes because of overcrowding and because the residents' immune systems couldn't fight the COVID. The numbers went up and up. Helpers did their best, but because they had so many old-timers to look after, they couldn't help being a carrier. Family members weren't allowed to visit. "It was a disgrace!" said some family members. Nurses and workers had been trying to get better conditions for years but were ignored. Not all care homes were affected the same, of course, and we watched the news daily for results. Records were kept and reports made every day by Dr. Henry. Records came in from around the world. Great. Britain was especially hard hit. Italy, Spain and the U.S.A. They were all in bad shape. The prime minister of England said that having the virus was the worst experience of his life. Fortunately, he was only 57 and able to survive. Borders between provinces and between countries remain closed to this day. Airline trips fell to a trickle and remain so to this day. We relied on face book and email. The elderly who didn't have the technology suffered most of all. Those who were "hip" had cell phones. I was left years behind but chugging along so I can leave this record for my fellow man.

Canadians were admonished to come home from wherever they were. The wise ones did just that. The others are stuck with the consequences in countries far away. Farm workers from Central America could no longer come to Canada to work. Those going home for Chinese New Year were another example. Those on holiday including one of my granddaughters and husband who had gone to Mexico had to go into quarantine for two weeks before they could go back to work which was certainly a loss of income. Every case was different but it was felt anyone out of the country was subject to contaminating those at home or at least have that possibility. Each case was different and there were no ways of testing whether they had the COVID or not at that time.

I wished that I were in Hawaii. My condo share had been paid, and I was just waiting for the reservation to my beautiful two-bedroom apartment in Waikiki. Tourists were told to stay home. No use moaning or groaning. I had grandiose ideas of going to Brigham Young University in Liaha but that fell to pieces. Perhaps I could have taken a course by computer but I'm not knowledgeable enough—not even half. We were told nothing was certain as to how long this pandemic would last.

The only thing left is to make a list. "What am I trying to do at home in Vancouver this spring 2020." It's only for me but if it helps, use it.

1. Look after myself. Forget about being lonely.

2. Look after the house. Buy a new Swiffer.

3. Keep in touch with the family.

4. Keep in touch with the extended family and friends by phone and email.

5. Watch church services on *Zoom*.

6. Write my stories (*Dorothy's Story, COVID-19, Mother's Real Estate Deals, Boston Marathon* 2013)—that should keep me busy.

7. Keep a record of COVID-19 for those in the future to read.

8. Learn Spanish. I've got the books. How hard can it be? I've been trying for years.

9. Gardening. My rhubarb is doing fine. The squirrels ate the tomatoes (both of them). The strawberries weren't in the right spot.

10. Go to the bank. Do better records. Pay off debts.

11. Buy groceries. Stay within budget.

12 Be thankful for all those who have been so kind to me.

13. Say my prayers. Read my scriptures. Pay my tithing first. The rest will look after itself.

14. Rest.

15. Try to pay something to all those charities who are asking for money. Keep Bill Gates and his wife in mind as a good example.

16. Answer e -mail and slow mail.

17. If something drops and I can't pick it up, forget about it.

18. Exercise. Maybe the most difficult of all. Being stuck in the house is hard on the health.

19. Have a saying for each day (e.g., "It's hard to heat a house with the door open." That's what my mother used to say).

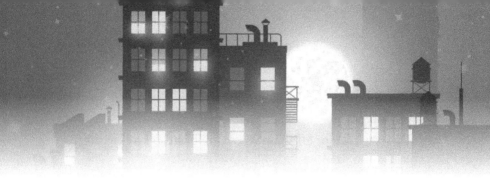

HOMELESS IN SEATTLE

loved that movie *Sleepless in Seattle*, but this is "Homeless in Seattle" and it seems like anywhere but Vancouver. Being a coastal city, they usually have the same problems as Vancouver—sometimes even worse. Apparently, the homeless population there is huge—far bigger than here in Vancouver, Canada. I wish I had the answer to them not having a place to live. It concerns me every day. I hate to see police involved. Someday, it may be one of them that's homeless. People on drugs, for instance, often need doctors, not police officers. The care given is quite different. Today, the police say that using drugs just has to stop. Where will they go? It will be civilians who have the expertise to help them. I think the police realize that. The fact that they are discussing places is a step in the right direction. The police are there to protect the laws of the land. It takes more when they are expected to be compassionate and understanding or to give an answer to the homeless problem. Pity.

Homes have several blocks in front of them. One is a healthcare system so that everyone can have medical attention. In Canada, my healthcare is covered, but my prescriptions are not.

Some people are covered, which is nice. Vitamins aren't covered, so I have to buy whatever I think I need. I try to buy the largest sizes so they'll last a long time. Other than that, I think I'm well cared for. In a Canadian's eyes, we feel sorry for Americans when we learn

16

that some family has had such huge medical bills that they lose their savings, their house, and possessions when they become sick and taken to the hospital, especially if they're self-employed. I know they'll say I'm wrong, and it's not mentioned on the news, but I've seen it happen to my American relatives.

On the other hand, they see me as getting free medical. Actually, nothing is actually free. We pay for it through taxes. I guess that's the reason the Americans don't want it. Please forgive me if I have said something out of place, but I know I'm not alone.

I love to watch the US News and the British news every night on Seattle TV. I would be so happy if the citizens down there would find a solution to homelessness. They seem to handle it the same way they do here. They kick them out of one place and then they have to look for another. That's not an answer. I have looked at it long and hard. You see, my grandparents and family gravitated to the Seattle area during the Great Depression or thereabouts and settled in the Monroe area. During the '30s, as my siblings grew old enough to work, some worked in the lettuce fields. Washington was one of the only states not hit devastatingly at that time. Many people look up to Washington State for leadership and thousands flock there.

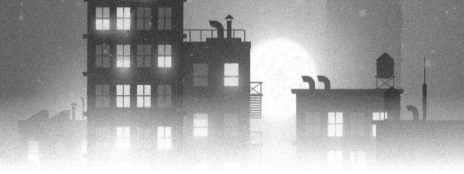

NEWS OF THE DAY

Distancing and wearing a mask, staying in fresh air if possible, washing your hands often, and staying away from people—not congregating in large numbers. All of these things are important if you don't want to get COVID-19 and perhaps die. Do not have visitors outside the immediate family. Do not travel. These are the things flashed across the nation, but sometimes it has fallen on deaf ears—especially in the beginning. It was as if everyone knew that Alaska had a tsunami but it didn't affect them, so why should they worry? Actually. Alaska did have a tsunami recently. It was on the news, but it apparently didn't cause much damage, so it was soon forgotten. The rules of COVID are forgotten at our own risk and that of everyone else's. Some restaurants closed. Some people were laid off from work. Schools closed. Some people were able to do work at home.

Some didn't think that COVID is even real. They don't want to wear masks or keep a two-meter distance from one another. They wanted life as before, going to restaurants and pubs at night, sitting side-by-side with their friends, continuing sports on the fields and on the rinks, taking their children to playgrounds.

They wanted Seniors to still share rooms with other patients and caregivers went about their chores, room to room. Children came to visit. Medics did their rounds until they found themselves with case after case of COVID-19 in the hospitals and people dying, especially the elderly in care homes. Even the provincial government didn't cancel the election. They did provide for spacing between each voter, which might have prevented more people from becoming contaminated.

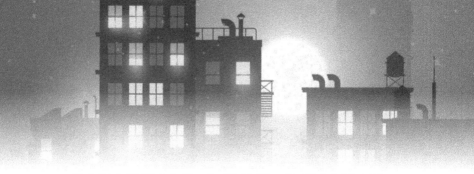

CITIZENS LEFT BEHIND

I came home to hear the phone ringing. It was my ex on the other end of the line, phoning from Mexico. He said, on one hand, he is frightened and on the other hand, lonely. I didn't know what to tell him. He had been dragging his feet since the beginning when the government gave every Canadian an ultimatum to come home. They had put quarantines on them within two weeks of lockdown. They were required to stay home for those two weeks to make sure they didn't have COVID-19.

My grandchildren, Leah and Ben, also happened to be down in Puerto Vallarta on a holiday, and when they came home to Alberta they had to stay in quarantine for fourteen days. They are back at work now, and everything seems normal but they both missed two-week wages.

When COVID-19 was discovered in Canada close to the end of February, the Canadian government was quick to realize the needs of its citizens, in particular special hospital wards.

With the focus on the loss of millions of jobs because of closing restaurants, offices and people working from home. Schoolchildren were now at home, and schools were closed.

Ottawa was quick to realize that many people rented or paid mortgages on their homes so they got assisted in their payments to keep families from losing their housing. If I'm correct, governments will want that money back when the crisis is over.

I forgot to mention that people that lost their jobs got compensation. The amounts were jaw-dropping, but it helped the economy. By magic you might say, $300.00 fell into my bank account. They also did other things for the economy and that was bringing down the bank rate; mine was down from 4.9percent to 3percent. I thought it was time to try to pay my line of credit down, as the higher rate was hard to bring the all-in-all balance was difficult to reduce. My interest last year was $18,000.00 interest, and my pensions were low. I felt I would have to find a way to decrease it.

The government in their wisdom (or lack thereof) had what savings we had in RRSP and RESPs made it necessary to use them all up by a certain age, so I have outlived what little I had. Nevertheless, by going on a really tight budget and paying the line of credit down as far as I can, I'll be glad I did. I haven't gone into malls unless absolutely necessary, and I'm trying not to use my MasterCard. However, things come along when least expected like the furnace and the huge roof. I mention it, so you might consider your own money matters.

I always used to give money to a number of charities but they seem to be hurting too, and I can't give like I used to. There are only two options. Spend less or earn more as the old saying goes.

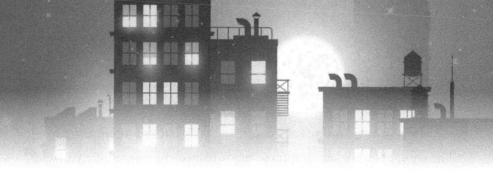

CLIMATE CHANGE

Everyone who reads this book could help with climate change. You'll have to if the world will ultimately change for the worse. Call it ignorance even if we don't. Your forefathers discovered oil and invented the automobile, the aeroplane, the radar, machinery, building materials—and you can add to the list. They were very clever to build trains, steamships, and bicycles. Did anyone suggest in the beginning that in doing so they were destroying our beautiful earth? So, you know what carbon dioxide looks like? Is it in your neighbourhood? Did you deplete a tree today? Let me take you on a visit to my neighbourhood.

For example, in my neighbourhood, before I was born, on every lot there grew tall evergreens up to the sky. Bears, mountain lions, and other creatures crawled in the woods, Squirrels filled the forests, eagles soared through the sky, and the rivers and streams were replete with fish. In the 1800s, many settlers wanted to come to Vancouver but the only way to get here was to sail around The Horn before there were trains. Then, Simon Fraser made his way clear across Canada by birch-bark canoe, turned around, and went back the same way he came, I believe. It was long and treacherous, and now, of course, we have long and treacherous freeways to look after.

Our lot was created after the time cars became popular and they needed a gas station/auto repair depot. Maybe you remember when the houses in Vancouver were all constructed with a garage in the back lane. Now "tiny houses" are replacing them. High-rises came before them, of course, but now too long ago the first one was built at the bottom of Granville Street but not to live in but as a commercial building, which could be seen for miles. Everything has been ascertained by city hall elected members and their thoughts on what the future should look like. As fellow citizens and neighbours, we complained because of parking problems, loss of sunlight, unpaved walkways and lanes, and general congestion. Without digging, I will only mention the carbon fallout. My table on the back porch was an oily black colour every day. I wiped it, and my lungs became plugged. I coughed and coughed. I couldn't say why. Then it got so I couldn't breathe. The few trees that were on the property across the lane where fourteen apartments were being built were cut down. Then COVID came along. Conditions were not good. Picture this happening. Actually, it improved things, as there were far fewer cars going to work every day and the units did get completed. The crows have even come back to some extent.

However, global warming is everything. That was only a sampling. However, the subject is gigantic. I'm sure I'm part of the problem. I *know* I'm part of the problem.

I have an automobile. It is energy efficient. Give me a plus. However, it requires gas. Give me a minus. It's not at zero. Since COVID-19, I have been confined to my home as much as possible. I'm not to use the car. Therefore, I have made rules. No shopping, sightseeing, travelling, visiting etc. Except grocery shopping, visiting the doctor and the pharmacist. Since March 1, 2020, I've only used approximately $33.00 in gasoline. Friends have helped. I sometimes go with my neighbour grocery shopping. My doctor is quite a distance away. I don't use the bus or sky train because of social distancing. I don't use a taxi very often, as it's expensive. I've postponed visiting because that's one way COVID is transferred from one person to another. Sad but true.

I gave up my nearly new car. It had taken me a full three years to pay for it, plus the down payment and insurance. Don't write to me giving your opinion on whether I should give up my car. I may be wrong, but I gave so much up to buy it and it was the only new car I ever owned. Otherwise, I never liked this new car from the beginning. It was built for someone else. to be sure. Every short woman would know it was built for a taller person. Visibility was a problem. The seat adjusted as my small frame required. Otherwise, it's admired by the young set, and according to the specs, it should be good for ten years or more. I think it has to be to get my money out of it.

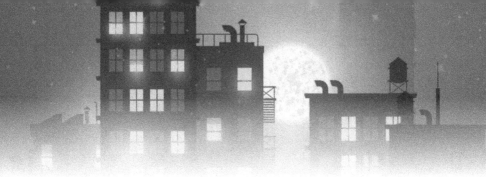

HALLOWEEN, 2020

COVID-19 is still with us. Dr. Bonny Murray is on the radio and TV with Dr. Dix every day to give us the statistics on the pandemic. British Columbia has a very good record right now. However, we have to do better so we don't slip back. Keep our distance-two metres. Let's stay within our bubble. Stay home, especially if you're over sixty. Don't attend concerts, beaches, shopping malls, tourist attractions, weddings, or church. Of course, if you're careful and wear your mask and everyone else does too, that would be helpful. It isn't a commandment but cautionary advice. It's all about the numbers, and if they go up, so will the rules.

It's easy to see there can be conflict. People are people. Life is built on families but it doesn't end there. Children want to play with other children. They learn from each other. Teenagers are very social. I always walked home the six blocks from high school with my girlfriend, whom I nicknamed Nylon. I worked nights at the Bolodrome with other teenage pin-sitters. Actually, the little ones aren't prone to COVID, but no one is sure of the future. We are cautioned to keep our hands clean by washing them often. Do you suppose children don't catch the disease because they have a bath every night? We surely don't know at this point. Playing in playgrounds with other children is also discouraged.

Eating out in restaurants is also forbidden unless distancing is enforced. Schools are closed.

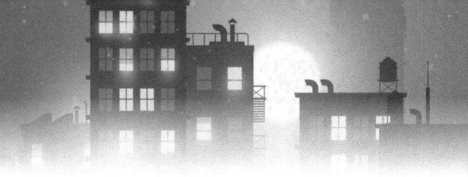

HAND WASHING, ISOLATION, MASKS
SANITATION, RULES, TRAVEL

O ver the next few weeks, the streets of Vancouver began to change. Dr. Bonny Henry spoke to us every day on CBC encouraging us to keep our hands clean by frequent washing and using antiseptic ointment to protect us from picking up germs. We were also asked to wear masks that covered our noses. I felt like I was about to rob the bank the first time I went in there, but I got used to it—sort of. We were to have a bubble of just those who were with us day-to-day. No shaking hands. No hugging acquaintances. Only those living in the same house. No large groups. And eventually, travel was discouraged. Taiwan was the first to close its borders, I believe, and they were rewarded for their effort but certainly not Canada and most of the world.

Early on, I got an email from Spencer, the son of one of my dearest friends. It said, among other things, that if you have parents or family in a nursing home to take them out. We were to find out soon how prophetic that was. Although it wasn't pleasant having to stay home most of the time, living all alone without my family even able to come to see me, I came to see how fortunate I still was.

Meanwhile, traffic got quieter somehow. Deserted streets. That still didn't stop prices from going up. Those wearing masks became more numerous, especially the Orientals on the streets coming and going to UBC or wherever. About 35 percent of the population is from the Orient, especially in Richmond. They are good neighbours but I think rather taken advantage of by the government. It's called The Empty Homes Tax. I can go almost anywhere else in the world and buy a house wherever I wanted especially when I wanted a place to go during the cold Canadian winter or a vacation home. For some reason unknown to me, the council cooked up a scheme to tax the owners of a home and left it vacant for any time, hence the name. I can attest that when China was about to take over Hong Kong in the eighties, the citizens saw the writing on the wall. Many sold their business and their real estate and made plans to move to a safe country elsewhere in the world, mainly Britain and Canada. I remember those days well, and so do the realtors of Vancouver who showed the houses for sale. They were sometimes able to brag about showing property in a good neighbourhood like West Vancouver, and when asked "Which one do you like?" the buyer would say, "We'll take both of them." We had two houses on the market at the time which had been on the market for a year with no nibbles. Suddenly, we had two offers within a week. The City of Vancouver must have been elated that year. No complaints whatsoever. The buyers were able to keep them in case things didn't go as China had promised when the agreement with Great Britain was made.

Some came over and tore the original house down and built a beauty in its place. Still, City Hall was happy, but they began to make unusual bylaws.

For instance, during the World Expo in Vancouver in 1987, the city tried to shut down the bed and breakfast rooms that were happily making room for visitors from around the world. With an extreme shortage of hotel rooms, people were sleeping as far away as Bellingham in Washington State and coming up for the day. The bed and breakfasts were a Godsend and made a lot of money for British Columbia. Tourists enjoyed meeting people and their great hospitality.

As another example, the city was wholly against what we called "in-law suites." Basically, it represented basement suites or very large houses the family could make room for a "mortgage helper." I personally was taken to court in Tsawwassen just outside the city because in our new house we had 2,700 square feet on the top floor and had developed the downstairs on the main floor. I was fined $1,500.00 for my offence in spite of the fact that in the Lower Mainland there was a vacancy rate of about 1 percent. They're still some of the highest prices I've heard of anywhere outside New York City.

That wasn't enough. After the expo, I was looking at houses in Dunbar, a section of Vancouver. I dabbled in real estate and was just looking and found that the workmen were filling the basement with dirt and gravel. I was astounded. They told me that the city had ordered them to do it because then no one could put a suite down there. "However, if you buy the house, you could easily dig it out." Yes, you guessed it. I didn't buy it.

What? You ask as if this had anything to do with COVID? Well, sometimes history repeats itself. In spite of the many negative things that you will learn about the pandemic, house sales are booming and were up 35 percent this year.

As far as the Empty Homes Taxes, I'm personally involved. I believe it started when, after living in Tsawwassen for twenty-five years, I put the house up for sale because my husband had died and I wasn't able to keep the garden up. I bought an apartment up the valley in Langley, and when that didn't work, I finally moved back into the house we had owned in Vancouver for many years. In the meantime, City Hall sent a form to my former address or whatever, and I never answered it. Then, suddenly, I got this bill for a humungous amount for Empty Home Tax. I was flabbergasted! I didn't have an empty house. Never had. I phoned around to my friends to ask what this was all about. One said that her friends were also having trouble with City Hall. They had an old house that was unoccupied, as it was only waiting for the wrecking ball to tear it down. It didn't even have an entrance to the front or back doors or steps to get into the place. I went down to Twelfth and Cambie where City Hall was located, and they told me I had to go to Victoria if I had a problem. I explained that I didn't have an empty house—never had one—and was not going to pay it.

They still send me a bill for more money than I receive in two years. I'm sure there are many more people in the same boat, COVID or no COVID. My friends had to sell their abandoned house and pay the Empty Home Tax. When COVID is over, I may have to get a good lawyer. Right now, I'm more or less confined to home.

How many times do we say "When COVID is over?" We all want to go on those vacations we're not permitted to take. We want to go shopping even if there's a sale and large crowds. We want to visit friends and have them over to the house. We want to see our grandchildren. I sure do. Mine live far away in Alberta. "When COVID is over," my son and daughter-in-law can visit me from 1,400 miles away. The border between us and the United States will be open again. We'll be able to go to Point Roberts and even through the main entrance at Blaine if there aren't the huge line-ups like we used to endure. We can fly to Hawaii.

Oh! How I miss Honolulu. Maybe I won't live that long, but if I do, maybe I can redeem that airline ticket Air France promised when I was in hospital two years ago.

I will never agree that anyone should pay an Empty Homes Tax on top of the tax they pay already. The Orientals in Canada have been abused enough. Those that came to Canada before the war were charged a head tax. I wonder who dreamed that one up when it was them that did all the donkey work on the railroads.

In the meantime, I'm comfortable in my hundred-year-old house. I live alone except for the Filipino family downstairs and the people upstairs. I say a century-old house though the sidewalks out front bear the date 1929—the year of my birth—with their many heaves and cracks on their journey down the street. The cracks are due to the gigantic firs in the boulevard along 24th between my house and the corner. I love those trees, which were probably here when the Musqueam Nations were the only ones in the neighbourhood. I pray that a huge storm doesn't send them bending in my direction. My husband and I bought the house in '66.

Maybe the city will take me to court. In Britain, a man's home is his castle. Apparently not in Vancouver. Since COVID, it's illegal to give your tenants notice, even if they can't pay their rent, and landlords can't raise their rents. I agree with that, but it can be difficult. My tenants have been here a long time, and I don't want them to leave. I decided I should help them instead. One thing you learn during COVID and that's to be flexible and innovative.

You hear the words, "We're all in this pandemic together." I accepted that and tried to find ways to do it. The first thing I thought of, as I'm not very inventive, is to save money on the electricity bill. I'll buy as many LED lights as needed and everyone can exchange their old bulbs. I've been doing that for a few years now but might have missed some. Hopefully, that will save us $60.00 a month with a bit of luck, which is my goal. I'm the worst waster I guess, so I decided to always wash my clothes in cold water and dry them on the patio whenever the weather is cooperative. I'll save twice that way. One because there is a saving in gas to heat the water and electricity to dry them in the dryer. There was a time when you weren't allowed to hang your clothes outside where the neighbours could see.

So far, I haven't given up watching TV. I love Knowledge Network and KTCS9. Those and, yes, the news. I never did like the murder mysteries much. They can go.

There's not much saving money if you don't have a goal as to where it should go. This keeps you on the right track. If we could save all together $720.00 or even less, I could send $20.00 each to a number of charities that ask me for money every year. There are approximately 9,500 charities in Canada and lots more in the States—and they all seem to have my address. I try to keep them happy, but it's become difficult. Gone are the days I used to comb the neighbourhood for the March of Dimes and be delighted if the lady of the house gave me anything more than $5.00 but even then, if five thousand people gave it helped those in need so I was happy, and all those mothers were happy as well. Now, of course, it's necessary to donate $20.00 or more to get a receipt for your income taxes. That's a good reason to give all you can or to choose your favourites. Some of you—maybe most of you—will understand when I tell you that a goat, yes, a goat and supplies for the charities' recipients now cost $200.00 or more. My son gave me that one Christmas, and I thought, *Fair enough*, and during COVID I didn't shop for presents for the family, so I gave him the same thing. Somewhere in Africa, we made some family happy, I'm sure.

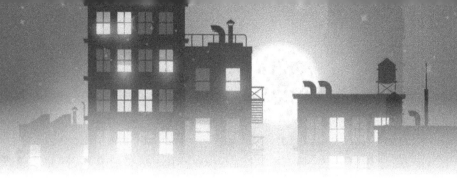

CHANGING TIMES

T here was a time not long ago when developers could give their tenants a two-month notice and come in, smarten the suite a bit, and re-rent it at a higher rent. I've known people to whom this has happened, and it's devastating, as they had lived there for years and never had plans on moving. That rule is curtailed, for now, I believe, so even good things can come of bad things. They're not homeless for now. Housing is expensive, so we don't know what their future will be.

People won't believe it but I know what it is to be homeless, though I never had to live in a tent. However, when my husband Bill was in the Navy and we had two small children, we were posted to Halifax. It was like Vancouver is now, having more people than places to rent so finding a place to live was extremely difficult. We ended up living in a wee log cabin in Melville Cove with no facilities. I'll never forget it. What does that have to do with COVID? Maybe nothing. Except, that particular winter, the children got the measles that they probably brought home from kindergarten. In some ways, it was like the COVID of today. The children could have been subject to lifetime consequences.

My sister Helene suffered from Shingles a throwback to chickenpox I believe. She was in a senior care home in Washington State before she died. She lived to be in her golden years, Health and playing Ten-pin

Bowling every week, but in the last years of her life, she feared running out of money, and if she did, they would move her to another care home which would offer far fewer comforts and might be far from her daughter who comes to visit her. She died before that fateful day came, but I wonder how much of it was attributed to worry. Many of us have the same troubles. Since COVID, I know living independently has its advantages and disadvantages. Some have no options. Myself, one of the unfortunate things about living alone is not having many computer skills. I chug along. I find it hard to do things electronically and bank business is rather hopeless when I can't go over to my branch and talk to the wonderful staff. I hire a university student part-time to help me with the computer and a single girl who helps me with many things in the office.

I always argued that I wouldn't be happy in an old folks home. First, I'm different than other people. I don't play Bingo and I don't drink tea or coffee or anything stronger, so I would be an oddball, I'm sure. The thought of living in a place where the women-to-men ratio is fifteen-to-one due to the fact of our men have died with all sorts of things over their lifetime like being killed while serving their country or in accidents at work—and even at play—and all sorts of things like being prone to liquor and smoking. I'm not saying we women don't die early sometimes, as they are the mothers of the world, but for reasons to be parsed by those far wiser than I, the result seems to even out that way. We loved them. They looked after us and loved us. And we miss them.

That said, I did go back to university last summer, and I went on the bus. My friend Hette was the only other senior of approximately forty students in a huge tiered room. The youngsters were taking the second-year English course, as a subject they all had to have regardless of the major. I remember taking it way back when, but my, how it had changed. I'd like to take more courses but COVID has certainly stalled most things. I tell people I don't even buy green bananas. They get the picture. Writing and reading keep my brain elastic, but it's a losing battle, I'm afraid. I find my pen slipping, and I'm falling asleep as I write and can't write coherently. In my mind, I hear Dr. Bonnie Henry whispering "Wash your hands, keep safe, and wear a mask." She is so inspiring that she is surely an angel. She's my angel anyway. I have tried to keep all her safety rules.

OCTOBER 2020

Will there be a time when the children will say, "What did great-grandma do during the pandemic?" Their mother will turn, amazed that the youngster knew anything about that part of history. "Well, I don't think she did anything."

Looking back, I notice that it's October and I'm still tied down more or less. What have I accomplished? More importantly, what would I have like to have done or still want to happen? It hasn't been dulled really, but getting from then to here may be difficult. You see "everlasting" is a very long time. We have different experiences, even in the very same minute—like seeing a hummingbird outside my window. It can't be, but I can't help thinking, *Is it one of those thousands of birds that were forced North from the fires this summer in California, Oregon, and Washington State?* Will this global warming make that kind of difference or will they find their way back South or perish here in October trying? I love birds and I wonder what the farmer's almanac predicted their future to be? Surely, they couldn't know that this was going to happen. All that grief from the loss of property unceasingly from week to week and to have British Columbia's forest escape but the other to be charred from stem-to-stern. Incredible that so many people were saved, having gotten out in the nick of time before their properties became a charred ruin. Tragic that anyone was lost and so sad the destruction fell upon the firemen volunteering to fight the blazes.

It reminds me of the winter of 1964 (If memory serves). After you read this, you may say there was no comparison. Actually, it was the exact opposite. Before you jump to conclusions read on:

The Christmas holidays loomed closer and closer. Here in Cloverdale, British Columbia, the children had finished their Christmas exams and I had taught my last day of school. Charlie had a job bricklaying on a Highrise in downtown Vancouver and it would soon be shut down until after New Year's Day. It was bitterly cold for Vancouver and snowy but what better time to go down to Chula Vista California and Disneyland to visit friends Lyn and Ed, and family. My mother was visiting us from Saskatchewan and had never been South, so what better time?

There would be Charlie, Grandma, Glenna, Maynard, and me—five in all. Douglas didn't want to come along with us. He felt his paper route was more important. No arguing would change his mind. That tells you a little bit about the boys looking back, I guess. Douglas was always conscientious, dependable, set in his ways. Maynard loved to travel, and when he was grown saw much of the world. Glenna was too young to have any say in the matter.

That Christmas would certainly be different. We all packed in anticipation. Our car was large as I recall—a nine-passenger Oldsmobile which was the pack horse of the family. The back was reserved for luggage and other essentials. I remember Glenna explaining later that she had to sit beside Little Grandma. As we headed south across the border, we were able to get into Oregon before nightfall. Slippery roads got worse hourly we peered through the window, looking for a place to stay on or near the I-5, but as darkness fell, we got anxious and felt any place would do. Nothing was familiar. We hadn't stopped to see my brothers and sisters in Monroe or Seattle as bad weather was in the forecast and we felt we were too many for anyone to look after. Looking back, I wish we had just gone that far and taken a motel but you know men drivers—always anxious to pile on as many miles as possible before dark.

By taking a turn-off south of Portland, we found a motel and were all thankful. Actually, the storm outside was so bad I didn't know where we stopped, but it was adequate.

The next day, the weather was no better, and after some discussion, it was decided to that we should veer off the I-5 and take the route along the coast highway where the roads would be clear with no ice and snow.

Bad decision but who were we to say? Maybe better had we stayed at home but who was to tell? It was further in a sense, but off we went. Hour after hour we travelled. The snow stopped, but the rain came down incessantly. Another thing everyone knows about men drivers is that they don't like to stop. We pressed on, and eventually, there were only flooded fields on either side of us. Cattle were trying their best to get out of the water by the hundreds. "That farmer should get out and look after that herd," I said. "Or they'll drown."

I felt so bad for those cows. "Where do they live? Where are their barns? Is anybody listening?" My husband just kept plodding through the rain.

Eventually, though, we arrived at a small village. I think you would say *town*, but it seemed small at first. Call it a "pause stop along the highway."

Everyone in the cramped car was ready for a stretch and a bite to eat. I can't recall a restaurant, but there was a store, so we went inside where we found a flutter of activity. We had noticed a number of Safeway truck lined up along the street as far as the eye could see and we quickly learned why they were all facing a southerly direction.

"The bridge is out ahead" was the answer to why these massive vehicles were facing in a southerly direction. "And probably won't be passable until tomorrow," was the consensus.

We could tell that mother was tired, and when she suggested we stay in the motel overnight (even though it was only a little past noon), we readily agreed, and Charlie headed that way while we shopped for groceries we might need. While doing so we noticed more and more travellers with the same idea as they crowded into the rather tiny grocery store by today's standards. Toilet paper and bread disappeared from the shelves like magic along with milk and dairy products, cans of soup, macaroni, bags of coffee, canned meat, fruit, and vegetables. It looked like the whole town was there loading up. We were saying to ourselves how glad we should be that the Safeway trucks were all there only to learn they were returning to Los Angeles from their northern run and were all empty. There was nothing going in that direction. Like us they had chosen the coast route. There was no other route south except for the I-5, which we had ignored to our peril. The adjacent road over the mountains was only a narrow road and no trucks going north this late in the day were getting through.

We were fortunate to get accommodations with a kitchen. Mother made lunch, and we all settled in. The pictures of the floods came across the front of the television, which was also provided. Those poor cows we had seen were now floating by, a frightful epic in front of our faces. By nightfall, almost all of the shelves in the meticulous grocery store were cleared of merchandise. All had been sold to residents and travellers headed south like us. It was quite a sight.

The bridge that we had just gone over north of there also had gone out, so even if we wanted to go back to Vancouver we couldn't.

We discussed what to do. We finally heard that there was no escape in the near future.

The next morning, the Red Cross was flown in and a church was opened up. Helicopters were flying people in and out but only to the next town. Charlie was commandeered as a guard for helicopters at night. I was called as a helper to the Red Cross to feed those that needed meals, both for residents and travellers.

The first morning, we made pancakes for those who came over to the church as we had flour, eggs, and baking powder, but later on in the week, the ingredients got worse and worse. Mother never did leave the motel but managed without their help. Eventually, when the store got supplies flown in, she was happy to have her tea and sugar. She was a pioneer from the prairie, so she wasn't too ruffled. Others were more inclined to become anxious and complained about the conditions. They just wanted to leave. Others who had four-wheel drive chose to go up over the mountain as soon as that trail was opened up. Some made it; some didn't and had to be rescued by the United States Army. Their cars were just left on the side of the road, which was only open to the south. The trail to the north was only open to the north and that was during the summer.

Others had their cars under guard until the helicopters could fly out but only to the next town, north or south. How they got home after that, I do not know. I surmised they lived there and were just in that town by chance.

Ten days passed, then eleven, twelve, when the United States Army started to bring in equipment to the mountain road to dig it out to a somewhat usable condition but they hadn't reached the town yet.

Believe it or not, we met some people we knew from Vancouver. They had managed to phone another couple that lived a little way from this town. The road was open between the two, and we were all invited to their house for supper one night. I'd say that was the highlight of the experience.

Christmas came and went. I really can't remember it. It was pretty meagre, I'm sure. No tree, no lights, no gifts, no scrumptious meal. However, we had a lot to be thankful for. We were safe.

We had a good place to stay. We had friends to visit (in a way). We had each other. We could even get letters mailed north and south to tell everyone we were okay. And, oh yes, we were on a list with about two hundred others to be led out of there as soon as they could get the road opened up over the mountains to the south. It must have been a rugged job for the Army volunteers, considering the snow and ice that had to be ploughed through, but finally, we were on the list with those that were still waiting to follow a truck out to freedom you might say. People still unable to leave were shocked to find that the Red Cross actually asked to be paid for their services. When it came to our turn, they said we didn't owe anything, as we had both volunteered and they had checked their records and found that we had contributed to the Red Cross that year. I was so happy, as I have always given to many charities and was indeed glad I had included the Red Cross on my list. It certainly wasn't a large amount, but I supported their worldwide support to those in need in my small way. All good things that go around come around.

We did have to agree with the rescuers that if our car broke down on the way that they would pick us up and push the car to the side of the road where we could pick it up in the spring. The thought was rather frightening but better than the alternative of staying in that tiny town away from home till the snow melted.

Early the next morning, we left with a huge line of cars before and after us (fore and aft as we would say in the navy), carefully following on a frosty narrow path upward and forward toward Southern California, still hours away but, above all, FREEDOM!

We were soon to learn what they meant by that ruling that if we got in trouble, the car would be left by the wayside when we saw the large number of cars, motor homes, camper vans, and so forth sticking out of snowbanks along the road.

"Will this journey never end?" came a voice from the back seat.

"Are there any washrooms?" came another.

Can you see why I might tell you about that incident? Can you see how having gone through that without feeling sorry for myself and having gotten through it with all the major disappointments was character-building? Can you see how it steeled us for anything our lives could throw at us? Well, *nearly* anything. If Charlie were here, he would say "COVID is a piece of cake. I lived through the blitz in London during the war."

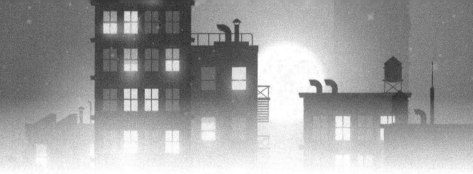

HOW WILL THE FUTURE
BE DIFFERENT?

COVID rather crept up on me. The first time it hit home was when the lady who takes me to church in her car told me that her brother back in China—the one who's a doctor—had been stricken by the pandemic. I was shocked, though I shouldn't have been. He was closest to the epicentre, but doctors are always protected, are they not? Apparently not. She was so worried, I didn't know what to say, but I worried about her. I also knew that her grown daughter was living over in London. The news of the pandemic was all ablaze with news around the world. Even Britain's prime minister, a young man of 57 and a new father, had been stricken. He said it was the worst thing he had ever experienced.

I began thinking of those nieces of mine in the Seattle area. I heard nothing much from them except a bit on Facebook. Washington State was the first to be hit and maybe one of the worst of any state in the US. When I thought about it, I figured that the residents there probably journeyed back and forth between the Orient more than those of any other state, as they were the closest to it. British Columbia could have been next, and I hope everyone was doing what Doctor Henry was telling us on CBC. "Wash your hands; stay home; stay two metres away from the next person; stay away from crowds, including beaches, shops, malls; and stay within your family." That was the gist of her message anyway. I thought I should obey. I certainly didn't want COVID.

It got worse. Many maps of states in the United States were broadcast with red dots, broadcasting the severity of the disease. Red dots in California, New York, the Eastern Seaboard, even Utah—I couldn't list all of them that were badly infected. We were all affected. Disaster loomed. Nurses complained about conditions in elderly care homes. They had wanted better conditions for years, but their voices hadn't been heard. Now, overcrowding came to the fore. Infection was rampant. Caregivers who were poorly paid were doing two or more jobs, and so the pandemic spread.

One day, I got an official-looking email from my friend Lil's (name changed) son Randy. Basically, among other warnings, it said that if we had any elderly parents in Care homes to get them out NOW. I may be repeating myself but I was impressed that he should send the information to me. Our families were always close, but he was in Ontario, and his immediate family was in Arizona and California. Surely the plague couldn't get to that desert state. I had a lot to learn.

I was thankful I was in my own home, but the message awakened me substantially, especially when the spec came in from North Vancouver, Ontario, and Quebec. Old folks were dying in considerable numbers—much higher than that of the rest of the population.

It wasn't difficult to realize I was one of those poor creatures. Apparently, we oldsters have weaker immune systems, and that leaves us vulnerable. I wondered too, did it help that I'd had an ordinary flue shot? I thought about it and wondered "Wouldn't it be a joke if I dodged COVID and died of pneumonia or any ordinary flu? At least I had lowered the odds by being vaccinated for the flu.

In care homes, they didn't even allow the families to visit. This disrupted families on both sides of the glass, even if the old-timers had dementia or Alzheimer's. It was wonderful to hear of people caring so much for their loved ones. I had rare visits to my mother, 1,400 miles away, and also my sister Dorothy's family. We had no father. We had an unwritten rule, however, and that was, "As you treat your parents, so will you be treated when you are old."

I remember the year before I was in the hospital, a trip to Portugal had been planned. I'd already bought the plane ticket with Air France, and it had to be postponed. Due to the circumstances, it was put in abeyance and is still recorded somewhere in the great beyond of unused tickets. Grandson Bill and his wife Delana were going with me, and eventually, that year they were able to go to Paris, but in a short while, I did get well enough to be released and had these lovely little ladies assigned a home service by Vancouver General Hospital to assist me with my bathing each morning for thirty days in a row. There was a little switch to it but looking back I enjoyed it all the same. Every morning around 10:00 or 11:00, one of these sweet little ladies would arrive to do her job. I had been up and had a shower at about 8 a.m. I really didn't need them as assigned, but with their mop and cloth, they did other household jobs, which I was thankful for, and I enjoyed their company. Thinking back to that time, had it been an epidemic, it would have been explosive, as every hour they went to a different assignment and could have caught COVID in their travels or passed it on. I wonder where they are today, as at the end of the assignment at the end of the thirty days, they disappeared as miraculously as they appeared. I often wondered if I got the service because, for years, I had given to the hospital foundation. I always felt that if I could help them purchase all the equipment they needed, it would be there if and when I needed it. In the meantime, hundreds of people would likely be glad it was there.

LONELINESS DURING
THE EPIDEMIC

Yes, I am lonely sometimes, but I'm one of the lucky ones. I'm really not alone. I have great renters upstairs and downstairs. During an epidemic, it's the little things that count. We have to stay apart to stay safe, but we look out for each other, and there is protection together. The first thing I decided was that we should not meet down in the laundry room, so I decided I could use my old machine and wash only on sunny days, as I don't have a dryer. It worked from March until October, but last night, I hit a wall. My lift isn't working but in the end, without asking Thimie downstairs, I figured it out and came and got my wet laundry out on the back porch, took it down, and dried it in the dryer. Perhaps a little thing but so important. She does many things for me besides working about seven days a week to keep herself and her two teenage children afloat. Come summer, I'll be able to hang the clothes on the back porch again—at least on sunny days. The people upstairs are always here to take in the mail and share a cheerful conversation.

Not having visitors is gross (as the kids would say) but necessary. I sat and knit six little bonnets for newborns until I ran out of wool. I contemplated doing some sewing, as the materials had been sitting around for years. Then, I realized that in moving here, one of the boxes went to Mission to my daughter's and the sewing machine came here.

46

That wouldn't do. The curtains I was going to make would have to wait. I watched a whole lot of television, finding KCTS9 on a regular basis. I saw Mr. Bates do the same program, helping the Blacks find their ancestry over and over again, which was fascinating. I know what it was to find my family and even began to think that my mother may have some black blood, as her complexion was dark and she avoided going in the sun. She never told us about her ancestry. I don't think she ever knew.

She was taken in by Jessie and Alexander Smith in Minnesota when she was about three years old. She's blessed with lovely curly dark hair—just like my sister Dorothy. I had straight blond hair, so who knows. Sometimes, I imagine Mr. Bates interviewing me on television and finding me related to Ken Maynard, the cowboy in the movies about in the '30s. Don't laugh. All the others he's interviewed were equally flabbergasted. My son, Douglas, found my birth father after spending hours on genealogy networks. I watched Knowledge Network but skipped the murder stories. CHEK TV had the best newscast, but with so much going on with the Donald Trump administration, how could I miss that? I also found BBC News, which kept in touch with the world. It never mattered how late the programs were on. I had nothing to go to bed for and nothing to get up for. I cleaned the house, and it looked pretty good for a while, but my greatest pleasure was keeping in touch with people by email. (Who invented Facebook anyway?) That or on the phone. My contract allowed me to phone across Canada, and I pay a little extra to include the United States and my relatives down there. They didn't include Hawaii for some reason. I was so happy when they took the first two digits away from the phone numbers like they had done in the States. The other great invention as far as I'm concerned is spellcheck. (Pause for laughter.)

47

My sister-in-law in Alberta said that she found herself sitting and watching the weather network. I figure that might be okay on the prairies, but here in British Columbia, it's pretty well the same as Seattle. Rain. Those fans who live down there are probably conscious of the fact that their weather forecasters are trying to make it look interesting.

Let's take a look at what I wrote down: Here I am sitting on a lonely COVID morning. I happened to turn on nonchalantly, you guessed it, the Weather Network. Believe me, it was so exciting watching things that are going on out there:

1. Florida. Sunshine, certainly wouldn't mind being there.

2. India. Terrible at Missisababa or someplace.

3. California. Still terrible fires. People are fleeing their homes with whatever they can carry in the truck.

4. Calgary. Snow. That's important to me with family & friends there. Accumulation on the foothills.

5. Podcast. I'm not sure what that is.

6. Advertisement. I could do without the ads. I don't need a car because I can't go anywhere.

7. Another ad. Gym classes. I can't go there either. Too many people.

8. Abbotsford. 12°C, etc.

9. Kelowna. About the same.

10. Whistler. 198 inches packed snow.

11. Vancouver. Boring

12. Weather network. Boring.

13. Prairies. Above freezing. Boring. Seasonal values.

14. We're hanging on. When will COVID end?

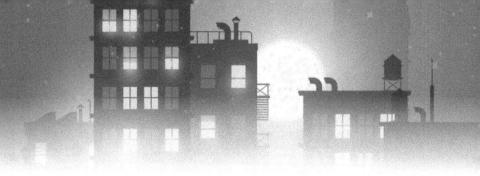

WEATHER CHANNEL

Hurricane Hazel took Toronto by surprise. Eighty-one lives lost. Many left homeless. *Toronto can't have tropical storms.* That's what people thought. Apparently, they can. They lost their bridges, and the Humber River rushed downhill. I lived near there as a teenager, so I remember it well, and now the weather network is saying it could happen again. I hope not.

And now the long-range forecast. Seasonal. Boring." I know you're not interested, but did you know the polar bears are really being affected by global warming? Now that's important. The poor bears are getting fewer and fewer. Soon they'll only be in books.

Compost made in two months. Kitchen waste to farmer's fields in two months. That's pretty interesting. Our wastes are always an important subject. Recently I heard we only recycle 13 percent of our waste.

That's the bad news.

My friend always sends her old clothes and those of her children back to the Philippines, which is about once a year. I have a closet full of clothes. They're pretty old-fashioned, but I still wear them. Waste not, want not.

Back to the weather news:

15. India. Horrible floods. A huge bus tipped over.

16 Utah, Colorado and other sections of California. Terrible fires.

17. Lethbridge where my son and family live. Ice Pellets.

18. Ajax, Ontario. A dog tested the water and left in a hurry. Reminds me of the black Labrador we used to have.

19. Ad. For flex seal. For your Floridian boat.

20. Ad. for Suburu. Buy now before they're all gone. I love that advertisement where the dog jumps in the boat and sails down the river nonchalantly as the people go after him and save him. That's for Suburu, I believe. If you're reading this book a hundred years from now, did we lose the polar bears or were we able to save them?

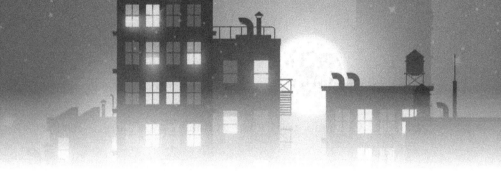

STARTING NOW AND
GOING BACK

I f this book had been a journal, it would be more organized. However, like my mind, it skips around a bit. The speeches by the parliamentarians are criticized, regarding what's been said and done, but I'm not in touch with what they've suggested in the past months. I'm treading in unknown waters, so I don't know . . . like the dog tasting the cold water. Yes, it's true that the Green party is important to the balance of power in British Columbia. In the past, it hasn't been shared too much for sure, but in a way, it makes them seem more important. It's a subject I would give in my writing class. Canada has an advantage in having several parties to choose from. Many think it's a poor time to call an election—amidst a pandemic.

My mother told me little about diseases as a child or what had come down through the family.

I found out that my mother had diphtheria as a child and had survived it. She was bow-legged from malnutrition, but we learned that the family had scarlet fever and that Doc Smith died in the hospital in Moose Jaw due to a broken jaw in 1918, the time of the Spanish flu that spread across the world. Isolation was the only defence against it—or so it seems looking back.

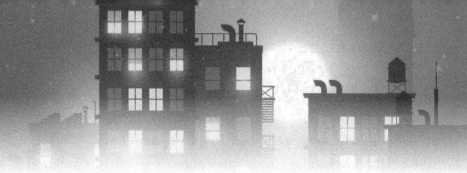

COST OF LIVING
DURING COVID

Since the election, the CCPA sent out a form with all kinds of questions. It seems rather inappropriate, and maybe you'll agree, looking back. "What is your biggest concern as a result of COVID-19? I would have to say "the care of seniors." Why? Because I'm a senior, of course. Actually, before I answered I wanted to know what they planned on doing. If I were twenty years old, I would probably say something different. I'm sure like jobs or education or student loan repayments asking what they've done and what they plan to do and when it will start. Will schools get proper ventilation? Will we be able to go to school, or will we have home school? Will we have to pay for any of our books?

As a senior, I might welcome extra money, of course, but seniors have a different need for every grain of sand on the beaches of Hawaii. However, they *could* be put into categories, I suppose. A sixty-seven-year-old will probably have fewer needs than a ninety-year-old: Maybe I could put down a few thoughts. I can't cover every single one.

Approaching sixty-seven years old. A newly retired person would probably have some savings—even some income tax returns—depending on what time of year they retired. Statistics say that the average person has little or no savings but if they've read this book, they will try to correct that by starting a savings plan by putting something aside every payday. Many will own their own home fully paid for if they had a twenty-year mortgage. (Just pay like the rent. You'll be glad.) They'll have some insurance, furniture, car, bicycle. Clothes, maybe a cottage or holiday lot . . . other assets, a spouse still working so you can combine earnings. Add your own or what you hope to have.

1. Approaching seventy years old. Maybe a part-time job. A hobby you just love that makes a little money. The rest is about the same.

2. Approaching seventy-five years old. At some time, you're required to spend your RRSPs and RESPs. They just seem to disappear. Gone too (maybe) is that Visa or MasterCard with the huge balance allowed. Too difficult to pay. It's dangerous, as you don't, under any circumstances, want to carry a balance due to high interest rates. In fact, you don't have control over any bank charges.

3. Approaching eighty years old. If you've lived a good life, things should be quite normal, but if one spouse is older, you just might outlive them. You'll be surprised how fast the money can evaporate. Death can be expensive. Of course, you're both going to live to be a hundred. I'm ninety-two, but I don't buy green bananas. My husband lived to be eighty-two.

4. Approaching ninety years old. Decide not to have the work of a house. You need a mortgage helper. Maybe you've always had one. That helps. RRSPs and RESPs have all gone due to legislation. Government pension plans are very small. They don't even pay the rent each month. I haven't been to a mall

in two years. Maybe it's time to go to a care home. It seems it costs five or six times the regular cost of accommodations if you can live on your own. Not everyone can. I don't have the magic, though I do live on my own. If you have a part-time job now, congratulations. If you have savings, it'll be hard to hang on to them. You may have to give up your car.

5. If you live to be one-hundred, you are to be congratulated. You will receive a letter from the queen, having survived all that life has thrown your way.

October 22, 2020

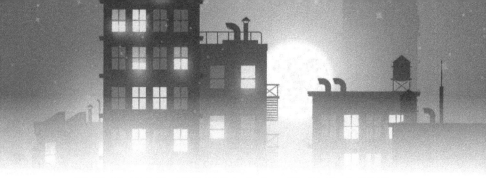

PRESIDENTIAL DEBATE

Resident Donald Trump and incumbent Joe Biden go at it like schoolchildren on the proverbial playground. President Trump seems to have no idea what should be done to defeat COVID-19. He feels that it will just go away and that there will be a vaccine for it within weeks. Considering the fact that it took years to find a vaccine for Polio, no one else seems to agree with him even, though there are physicists around the world trying just that. Nothing that's available has worked so far, but he brags about how little he had to pay on income taxes and says it's because he's smart. In truth, he's remodelling a run-down hotel and gets grants from the government. In a time that Black Americans are trying to get freedom and acceptance, he talked about there not being enough jails. In the time of Black Lives Matter, he calls the Mexicans "rapists." He has given orders to keep building the fence between the United States and Mexico to keep the Mexicans out, and he has little respect for ending global warming—or so it seems. He also feels that the voting poles have been tampered with and that is the reason he hasn't won. A recount showed differently.

My notes are poor perhaps, but Joe Biden replied "Science over fiction," signalling his support for clean energy and healthcare reform. Donald Trump separated children from their parents, and after all this time, they don't know where to find them. It's so sad! There are many

Latinos in the US, and I imagine they have fears of voting. Joe Biden hopes to secure citizenship for them.

Being Canadian, I'm just an onlooker, but many Americans are as shocked as I am by Trump's behaviour. However, there are many Americans that follow everything he says on Twitter every day. Many don't understand how beneficial healthcare would be for the whole nation, and many have a terrible view of the Blacks. Many are killed every month by the police, and many Latinos are lost trying to get away from horrid conditions in Latin American countries. They also have many deaths because of COVID-19. However, their numbers are not broadcast where I can see them. However, news seeps in through the BBC and other broadcasters. Italy's situation was so bad for a while that they were on the news every day. Spain also.

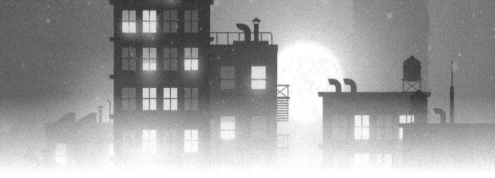

PLAN OF ACTION

Always keep global warming in mind. This hundred-year-old house needed double-thick windows when we bought it years ago in 1966. People in our life—even workmen—said, "Don't update it. It will take years of savings in heat to pay the money back." Nevertheless, we changed the windows, not only for ourselves but for the planet. Yes, even that long ago, there were some of us not using the name global warming but nonetheless economizing our resources. Not only did it pay itself back in three years in heat savings, but we were amazed by how much quieter the street noises were. Since then, we have never hesitated. It was the right choice. Our latest upgrade was the eleven-year-old heating system. Next, it was the roof that needed replacing.

It too will be costly but worthwhile. (The roof was replaced in December 2020.) Better for us. Better for insurance. Better for the planet. When the workmen got up there to work, they found that underneath they found that plywood hadn't even been invented yet when this house was built.

"Many of life's failures are people who did not realize how close they were to success when they gave up." Guess who said that. Thomas E. Edison. Don't step on anyone's toes to get where you're going. Love everybody. Want everything you have for everyone else. Sounds impossible. How do we do it?

We work and pay income taxes. If we earn a lot, basically, we pay a lot. If you're happy with that, you'll be a happy person. We buy stuff, and we pay tax on that as well. Buy a new fridge; you pay a lot but you are thankful you can buy such a beautiful appliance for your kitchen. You realize that your country has many things requiring money, especially to prevent global warming. You get in trouble if you overspend, especially on your credit card.

You're also the guardian of your own money and must handle it with care in case of disasters, droughts, floods, or even a pandemic in the future. All of these things have happened in my lifetime, believe it or not, including war and the Great Depression. Believe me, I never expected a pandemic. However, my experiences haven't trained me to depend on anyone since I was a child, although, in a sense, we all depend on each other. Perhaps I've done some things right and helped others along the way.

Getting back to the pandemic, no one saw it coming. Had they, we may have done things better. We must be thankful for what was done and done well. As they say, "We'll get through this." In the meantime, we have medical protection and help for everyone, which will contribute to as quick of end to COVID-19 as possible. We won't have the troubles other countries are having, and if we do simple things like staying two metres away from each other (no that's not easy), wear our masks, wash often, get vaccinated, report if you have symptoms etc., we shouldn't have the troubles that other countries are experiencing. There have already been many infections, many hospitalizations, many deaths, and many countries unable to cope. We're social creatures, so if we disobey, we may not be charged, but there will be a price to pay by someone or many parties. We have weddings, funerals, musicals, dancing, and sports games. Also, it's imperative that we wear a mask when we have to go out in public. Some say "Nobody can tell me what to do." Wrong attitude. COVID-19 can gallop among these people. Others say "How long must we stay separated?"

I wish I knew but the answer is "As long as it takes." I haven't heard it addressed but the doctors in charge let us know the casualties just about every day and also how the pandemic is trending. If the hospitals get overloaded, there's no hope. New Zealand reports that they're doing well, but they can't let their guard down. Taiwan closed their borders as soon as it realized what had happened, and they have very few cases.

Canada has had to keep its borders closed and only let Canadian citizens back into the country with quarantines in place. Considering that the USA. is only a few miles away, this is a step that hasn't been taken lightly. Airlines have cut most flights. I've heard figures like 90 percent bandied around.

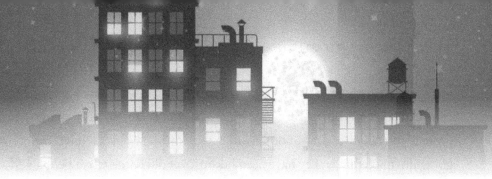

HOUSING

Some years ago—so long ago I can barely remember—the government in the United States was giving anyone a deal if they would take on fixing up run-down properties in places like Detroit—sort of like the fixer-uppers on television today. Fix it and list it. I never took them up on the offer, but those who did must have helped a lot of people. Everyone involved gained. Finally, in my experience, there was a time right here on the lower mainland when there was row upon row of houses that were started but left unfinished. The builders had gone bankrupt. I don't remember the particulars, but neither the banks nor anyone else could help them. I guess they didn't see the future and just let them go to the wind like the dirty thirties all over again. My husband and I didn't have much money, but he was a bricklayer and was willing to try buying one of these shells and finishing it. Each weekend, we would work on it with the help of local tradesmen. In the end, we couldn't sell it, so eventually, we decided there was nothing to do but rent it. At the last moment, the bank agreed to mortgage it to a young couple, and everyone was happy. There were many people who wanted the house, but the banks wouldn't give them a mortgage.

Today, there are so many people living in tents in areas of the city—usually in close proximity to grocery stores. From time to time, even throughout COVID, the authorities remove these "campers" by force and they move to wherever they can find streets, parks, or empty commercial lots. There isn't anywhere else for them, so this causes great inconvenience and another order to move. I'll have to give the government credit, as they have been taking over old hotels to get people off the streets, but Vancouver, having the warmest winters in Canada more or less, seems to be the only place to be where they wouldn't freeze to death during the cold weather. There aren't enough places to go, and the spaces are hardly what anyone would want as permanent housing. It seems to be an unending problem, and of course, with so many people losing their jobs because of COVID, it's an aggravation for sure. Affordable housing is number one on the list. That doesn't seem to be happening. It's not easy, but it is absolutely essential. Being old, I lived through the war. Whatever rules they had at that time, they certainly didn't seem to be working. My mother and sister and I arrived in Vancouver and the tourist places that they had at that time were single-room places near English Bay with a hot plate. These places have been lost to high rises, which are expensive. Very expensive, indeed, on the world market.

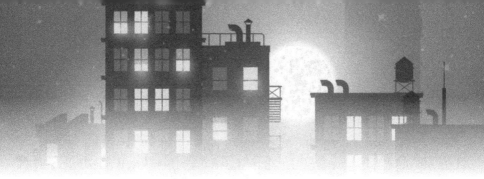

COST OF LIVING

Being elderly, I have a lift to get upstairs. However, it doesn't work very well. The workman who came to fix it charged me $500.00 for one hour's work. A month later, he came back again, as it was not working again. Another $500.00. He replaced the board and put it under warranty. And yes, this third month, it isn't working. Ever been caught in a lift? Well, it's kind of scary. I can walk up the stairs as long as I don't have to bring up my walker or armfuls of groceries. Another worker came to fix it this time. He only charged me $250.00, but by this time, I was fed up, and the next time it broke down, I decided, though inconvenient, I would make it up the stairs or just stay home until he comes back on his own and fixes it for good.

Other prices are also going up, though it may be gradual. Millions were left without jobs because of COVID. They also had little saved for a rainy day. Fortunately, we all have healthcare, but some people like me have a pension of $1300.00 and probably don't get their meds paid for. Mine cost approximately $170.00 per month. I sometimes skip a dose or two at my peril (if it's close to payday) and buy a three-month supply to save by avoiding pharmacist fees. I do recommend the latter but I don't recommend ever missing your daily dose.

Senior housing is often $1.000.00 to $7.000.00 per person in care homes. The rates could even be higher, whatever the traffic can bear. The advantage is that no one will be refused housing. The bad part is that you may be put on a long waiting list to get in. The death rate under COVID was the highest percentage in the country, for protection, visitors weren't allowed, month in or month out. It was terribly depressing for families that like to visit their loved ones in care. I'm fortunate; at ninety-two, I'm still living independently. With all of its problems, I prefer it.

Another disadvantage about care homes as I see it is that people often have to share rooms. Therefore, besides other disadvantages, if one gets sick, it's likely for the other residents to be infected, too. Nurses and caregivers are also poorly paid. They were already fighting for better wages way before this happened. Perhaps doctors were also fighting for better conditions, which were slow in coming. Many helpers also worked in more than one place during the day to make ends meet. This was contagious as well and, as you can imagine, terribly dangerous.

What's worse is, at any age, living in a tent city. It must be terrible with just a porta-potty, no showers, no heat, too hot in the summer, too cold in the winter—freezing cold, in fact—and no choice of neighbours. But the worst thing of course is being forced by the police to move. When asked "Where to?" to get the answer "Anywhere, but not in my back yard."

People say to me, "Well you don't know anything about it. You're rich! Yes, in a way I am. The rich don't think I'm rich, but they don't care. I didn't start out rich. The first place I remember living in was a one-room place across the tracks on Cornwall Street in Regina, Saskatchewan, with my mother and sister in the middle of the Great Depression. We went from one house to another—no furniture. Once, I remember a wooden orange box in the corner on Victoria and Albert Street, but I never felt like we were poor.

On CBC this morning, they referenced people (namely, refugee families) who have become displaced and have had to go through far worse than I have had to face—with COVID-19 to boot.

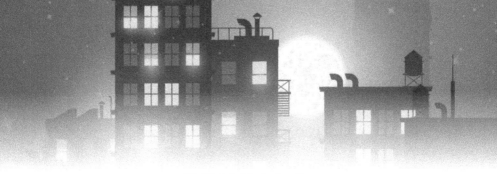

RENTALS

Pretend you're a homeless family looking for a rental in Vancouver or perhaps elsewhere on October 22, 2020.

1. You really didn't have the money for that expensive of a rental.

2. As a landlord, I know they can find all kinds of excuses if they're fussy about who they rent to—especially at this time when there are shortages of space and many to fill them. In Vancouver, for as long as I can remember, there has been a 1 percent vacancy rate. That's about as close to zero as you can get.

3. There are reasons for the shortages. Long wait lists for construction permits. Lack of space. Vancouver can never get bigger. It isn't like the prairies where you might be able to build more if willing to eat up on prairie land.

Therefore, the cost of land in Vancouver requires tearing down a building before putting another one up. Destruction of greenery. (That's what makes Vancouver so beautiful.) Building costs. Import costs. Cost of wood. Destruction of forests.

Labour costs will be higher, and the list goes on. Everyone wants to live in Vancouver, as it has some of the finest weather conditions in Canada.

I wish I could tell you the elected councillors in city hall have big plans to put up affordable housing, but now you see why they may not succeed, including the "Not in my backyard attitude." If such plans were in the works and I thought they were doable, I would list them right here.

Instead, I'll go back to 1939 when I first arrived here. I feel so sad for those who have no place to live. Don't quote me, but there are thousands of singles—some in tents, some in empty vehicles—with nothing to their names. So, this is the most important thing on the agenda in my eyes. I could be wrong. I shall let you decide.

Our mother had saved for two years to pay our way from Regina, Saskatchewan, to Vancouver. I think the tickets were $10.00 each to go in an old-fashioned car dated in the '20s or '30s at best—color: "as long as it's black," as the saying used to be. Of course, she needed expense money when we got there and for a place to sleep along the way. When we arrived, we went to the usual tourist place—a one-room with a gas grill and a bathroom down the hall. It was located in beautiful English Bay.

There were few hotels at that time.

It was four years after the workers who were working for fifty cents a day in work camps had finally had enough and congregated at the post office to plan a trip to Ottawa on the empty train cars to complain about the conditions. However, the trip was very dangerous, and by the time they got to Regina, the RCMP and city police were told to stop them. My little sister, who was about four years old, and I witnessed it that day and asked our mother what they were doing as they came right between the house where we lived and the one next door. My mother told us they were looking for sticks to defend themselves with.

Getting back to Vancouver, there was a big building boom prior to the '30s but little during the depression—with the exception of one high-rise commercial building at the foot of Granville Street and Stanley Park, along with a new bridge, both built with private money. Oh yes, and the City Hall on 12th Ave. It took the beginning of the Second World War on September 3, 1939, to change their working conditions and unions thereafter.

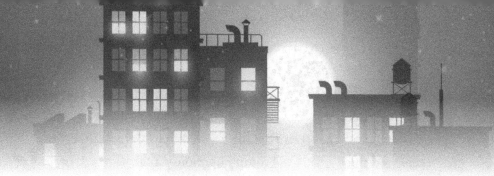

NEWS ACROSS THE BORDER

President Donald Trump's words will probably be repeated from now until forever, and his words on COVID-19 at this time will be no exception. First of all, he thinks that "COVID-19 will just go away by itself and a vaccine will appear within weeks." He gets very little agreement from other leaders, including Joe Biden, who will be his opponent in the primary. The population of the fifty states tends to agree with him, and they follow everything, he says on Twitter. I so wish he was right, but I lean on what history has proven when pandemics spread across the world; they can last for years and years. Doctors and scientists are working 24/7 to try and find a vaccine that will work, plus test it, produce enough of it to cover the population of the earth, provide facilities to apply it, provide the bottles to ship it in, and get doses to the majority of the population.

Some predict it may take years. Those who are older and are most vulnerable, incidentally, remember how long it was before a vaccine was found for Polio. President Trump thinks they will have a vaccine in a month or two. Therefore, he doesn't agree with those who caution us to stay quarantined and out of reach of others, clean our skin often, wear a mask when we're in public, and most importantly, not to travel, as that's the way this virus spread around the world. Everyone is vulnerable.

Of course, those who follow President Trump are prone to not following the rules that can save their lives and the lives of others around them, and they're still going to weddings, large dinner get-togethers, and pubs. Donald Trump's opinion is that it may all calm down when winter arrives. Opponents want the world to know that people indoors during the winter are most susceptible. Living tightly together is also a threat.

Trump's thoughts: "Success will bring us together." Biden: "Science over fiction." He also speaks about clean energy for the world. Election day is just around the corner. Joe Biden is against the lack of healthcare for everybody. AOC plan, not agreeing to the plan. They don't want to spend the money to halt global warming. Fracking is also a touchy situation and destroying the land.

As a Canadian in a sense, I don't have a say in what goes on in the US. I can't sit back, though, and not feel great grief over all the Latino children being taken away from their mothers who tried to bring them across the border into the States to escape the terrible troubles they are having in Latin America. As a mother and a grandmother, I mourn them and pray that Mr. Trump will not be re-elected in November and that the children will be returned to their parents and that the building of the wall between the United States and Mexico will stop. If Donald Trump is re-elected, maybe a wall will be built between Canada and the U.S. Since COVID, of course, the border is closed to unimportant crossings of the border between our two borders, but that's to stop the disease. The short time it was open proved disastrous. Vancouver Island had almost no COVID pandemic. US citizens said they were heading to Alaska, but in reality, they were taking a holiday in Victoria, British Columbia, and their numbers of COVID went up. Therefore, the border had to be closed to save the lives of those on the island. We're all waiting for the vaccine on both sides of the border so it can be opened again.

BECOMING A MILLIONAIRE DURING A PANDEMIC

You may have heard that many people will become millionaires during this pandemic. The rest of us will shake our heads and say "Impossible."

Were you amazed how many products started appearing on the Internet lately? Don't you wish you had thought of something like that? You still could.

What if you decided to include mailing costs? They may beat down the door to include you, so to speak. An interesting thing happened already. I never imagined it being possible, but some homes sold for 35 percent higher than last year in Vancouver. Houses are already a million dollars or more. Much more.

Food delivery. We didn't have Uber a few years ago. Now they even deliver food. Good idea.

What if you accidentally found an answer to cure COVID-19? Imagine being one of the scientists.

A new way to deliver information or just cheaper? Mail rates are outrageous! Wouldn't you make certain people very happy? Did you ever think you'd never use a letter but found great message devices on the internet? I can't even get out to post a letter or get to the bank. Yes, other answers are on the way. I may not agree with them, but many do.

BELLE MAYNARD CURD

Every single day offers something to be thankful for on this side of the fence as the saying goes. Love others. Be thankful to your Savior. Forgive others, although it can be difficult. Smile when you don't feel like smiling. Wayne Gretzky, the most famous hockey player who came from the Edmonton Eskimos (name to be changed shortly) was a great model for all of us. Somewhere, I read that growing up he learned:

1. To prepare.
2. To work hard.
3. To motivate yourself.
4. To visualize your goal.
5. To create an environment to make it happen.

He might add if you saw him today that, yes, these tenets still apply during COVID—*especially* during COVID or while facing any other problems that may come your way.

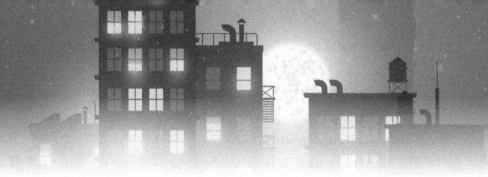

STARTING A BUSINESS

This may be the time to start a business. I think about it every day, and over the years, I have started businesses that seemed worth trying, and though there were only a few ventures that made money, I always learned a lot. Therefore, I wouldn't say I was a failure. I made money for the distributors, but in the end, it wasn't what I was looking for. I turned down many chances (they're all around, as the saying goes). They're just waiting to be discovered. I took courses, returning to university during the summer. However, I learned that good jobs don't usually come looking for you but be prepared in case that day comes along. Work at everything you love. Small amounts can multiply. Read a lot, study a lot, take courses and a language or two. One of the most important life hacks for any entrepreneur is a morning routine that gets your day off to a good start. Find yours and stick with it is—that's the saying that kind of tells it all. Some people knew what they were going to be since they were very young.

Don't put off starting a business just because of COVID-19 or going on a trip. I was all set to go to Hawaii last year (you put in your own destination). We could have gone, but for some reason, I didn't get there—maybe because my grandchildren couldn't go with me or maybe that was the time I ended up in the hospital or maybe because I couldn't get a reservation for the time I wanted. Now it's too late. Do what you need to do or want to do before you can't do it.

We are more likely to only notice the negative things like how many people have caught the disease, the hospitals overflowing, people dying, and the plague spreading.

The authorities used various methods to mitigate the damage. Restaurants had to close or move to tables on the street; seats had to remain two meters apart. Other restaurants closed entirely, and schools closed as well. Older grades went to computers at home.

Companies closed down or staff worked from home or started up on the net. Some people sold their homes. Strangely enough, realty prices held; in fact, they increased as there were many looking for a place to live. Probably a decrease in building brought this on. I had noticed very little construction going on, with few apartments but not many wanting to downsize.

There were no incentives to build that I knew of and no carrots for the common man to buy rather than rent. The building trades hadn't shut down and weren't part of the problem. Habitat For Humanity had been held back for years in Richmond it appeared for permits. I gave donations to Habitat, but I'm a very small potato, so I don't know the whole story. I had tried to buy a house in Alberta but the banks were difficult to deal with, me being at such a great distance. Perhaps they had been spoiled for too long and hadn't faced real life. They seemed to be waiting for the oil millions to come back.

Actually, we all should have started years before, but who would have known what the problems would be? I'm not complaining; it was no different. I didn't see it coming. I didn't take action. I didn't ever have a seventy-two-hour kit. I didn't see the mass poverty that could happen. The government spent a great deal of money to see that there were some safeguards in place. Of course, there were many complaints, but it seemed to help many recipients. Time will tell if it helped unemployment figures to stabilize.

In my own life, I remember my mother didn't want to go into an old folks' home unless she had her own room. If they had done that one thing with all the elderly, lives might have been saved this year during COVID. Many lives.

More recently, health helpers and nurses let it be widely known that they needed more wages. As a result, our staff were working overtime and working full time in one institution and then going to another institution to put in more hours to increase their income. This, too, caused the spread of COVID-19 and many more deaths.

The procurement of hospital and medical supplies for a disease that was never going to happen—not in our lifetime it was thought—wasn't an easy sell either, though the wisest amongst us foretold this long ago. However, there was an extreme shortage of medicine and supplies. Only the time when it would happen was unknown. Therefore, there was a scramble for meds and medical supplies. It was flying off the shelves at the beginning of the pandemic when the toilet paper and many other things disappeared from the stores just as they had in California.

Another problem was this: "If school started up, what would be a good class size in order to keep the children separated?" Desk plans were changed to accommodate the smaller class sizes.

However, keeping the distance takes a lot of teachers. The problems seem to come when the unexpected happens. From the outside where I am, I just can't imagine it. Years ago, I substitute-taught for a school in Surrey, British Columbia. It's a sad story, but two teachers from the school had gone up to King George Highway perhaps to pay a bill or go shopping or whatever (I was never told the purpose of their trip). I was eating lunch when the telephone rang and I was asked if I could take over a grade-one class for the rest of the year starting that very afternoon. The voice on the other end of the line seemed so desperate, I headed over to Surrey as fast as I could. It appeared that they had been crossing the highway at the light when a car hit one of them and she was killed. It was so sad.

I hurried over in spite of the fact that my classes at UBC hadn't aimed at any of the lower grades and there were forty unhappy children awaiting me. They were little darlings and Surrey was growing so fast that all the classes were overflowing. I shuddered to wonder how I could replace that wonderful teacher, but I would do my best to follow the guidelines. It wasn't like it would be today when I would have been given a helper. I still think of those children and wonder how they all turned out.

I can't imagine what it would be like if a pandemic had come along that year.

The university classes were mainly put on the Internet—or so I've heard. I would surely fail if that were me. I always wanted to write about my own classes in the '50s and '60s compared to now. We'll have to be patient. Stranger things have happened.

Before you say that ninety years old is too late to go to university, I have to admit I was the oldest to take a second-year English class, but I loved every moment. Not only have the teachers gotten a lot younger but they have moved the English building. The bus still goes up there, but the route has changed. I used to sleep in literature class. There I would be on a Saturday afternoon in the Army barracks, where it was so warm and so lacking in fresh air—not to mention probably I had been out to a movie the night before and hadn't gotten a lot of sleep. My marks were so-so.

A DIRE NEED

When cooped up at home for days on end, you get the queerest notions. Mine took the form of the following:

Looking after my possibilities of perhaps owning another property at my age is perhaps silly for an old lady. I guess it could be interesting but most would say, "You're too old," and would wonder why I'd want to do such a thing. I agree. I tell people I don't even buy green bananas. You get the point. Even with a down payment, I couldn't get a mortgage, and if I did, I would probably have a hard time making the payments. See what COVID has done to me. However, it hasn't deterred me from thinking of the homeless. Thousands depend on someone (or lots of someones) to help them. I would say it should have started years ago—long before COVID.

First of all, we should give it a name. How does "Living 24/7" sound? I thought so. Let's leave it for now.

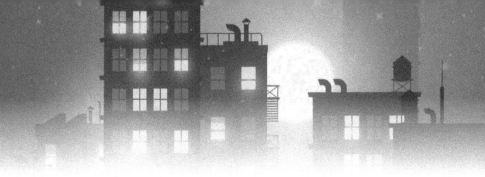

WAY BACK WHEN

L ooking back to my school days, I remember home economics as a great subject. My preserved pears were so perfect, the teacher entered them into the Regina exhibition. I was so proud of that. I also had my handwriting entered another year (cursive, of course) called the McLean's style of writing. Now I understand cursive writing is seldom read in school, never mind written. Preserving food in jars also wasn't encouraged, but it's coming back during COVID—even doing our own gardening. We had gotten used to canned goods and a refrigerator with a freezer attached for frozen goods. I must admit I still preserve beet pickles almost as well as my mother did when we lived in one room and only had a coal oil stove. It's one way of having beets every day if you want them, and they're so good for you.

Boil beets for approximately 2.5 hours; cool, peel, and slice the beets; then, place them in a sterilized jar. Add apple-cider vinegar that has been boiled with half a portion of water, ¼ cup of sugar, a little salt, and 1 tsp. cinnamon (all ingredients approximate).

I also make apple sauce. Certain apples are better than others.

Cranberry sauce from the package, cooked or uncooked. I like that too.

Rhubarb is delicious, too. If you don't have any in the backyard, find someone who does and get a cutting in the fall. Start your own garden wherever you are.

When the pandemic started, people got back to making bread and other baked goods, including cinnamon buns, cookies etc. Some are even making a business out of it or got work in a bakery. Some baked for shut-in family and friends. They couldn't stop to visit but it let them know they were thought of. We all need to be creative during a pandemic—well, anytime really. You will note that if you're determined, the use of tins and cardboard will go down, so you're contributing to helping protect the world from global warming. It may not seem like much in the grand scheme of things, but you'd be surprised.

A PEEK AT THE FUTURE

Since my school days, there have been so many changes, I couldn't recognize teaching methods at school. Looking back on COVID, there need to be changes beyond the last hundred years, perhaps a step backward to go forward. However, no ideas should be discouraged, ignored, or laughed at.

It could be a way to help the poor and homeless while enhancing the middle class. Note: I didn't say "decrease the rich," which I hear over and over again. As an example, I often hear that it's all the fault of the rich or the government or the police or the bankers or some other nation.

I'd like to give you a small example that happened to me rather recently:

It was the Saturday of the collections for the food bank. All the volunteers did their routes in their cars and drove to the ward church building to sort and prepare for the food bank pickup. It was November here in the Vancouver area, cold and raining cats and dogs as only the Lower Mainland can. I had unloaded my donation of groceries and was helping sort so they would be organized when the big trucks arrived from headquarters. Many others were working in the large auditorium. My bag of food was small, so I was there to give a donation because I had heard that the food bank could use the money more economically than we could at the food market. A young man, probably in his late thirties, was working beside me, helping with all the heavy lifting. I don't know how it occurred, but we started talking about buying houses. I learned he was living on subsistence, looking for a job, and he complained that he could never buy a house. I felt sorry for him and asked how much a house would cost. He told me a price and I had to agree with him. I lowered the price he mentioned. He answered, "Still too high." I lowered it to $100,000. He said, "Still too high." Then, I said $30,000. He said, "Still too high." Actually, that was the down payment for a first-time buyer's purchase; it came with a lot of government nuances, but from then on, you could own a house, just paying rent. He won the argument, though. It is tough.

People used to come to me for advice, including my dentist's secretary. While in the office, she asked me if she should buy an apartment on English Bay. They were large and beautiful. They cost $10,000, so you can see that this was a very long time ago. At that time, a house could be bought at about the same price (not as new, of course, and not in as good a neighbourhood). I didn't know what to advise her, as she would surely let me know if I was wrong. Instead, I asked her if her rent went up every year. She said, "It sure does."

"Well, maybe you should." End of conversation. I don't know if she bought one of those suites, but if she didn't take the chance, she missed out on a great buy. Those apartments today could not be bought for a million dollars.

One more example. This one is from more modern times. A friend of mine has lived in a two-bedroom apartment for many years in a great neighbourhood. Her rent went up from time to time, but the going price is now much higher than she pays. Recently, the owners of the building have told her they were going to take possession of the whole building and everyone would have to move. During all those years, she had never been able to put aside money to enable her to buy another apartment. Pity. She doesn't know where she will go.

I could give you many more examples but you get the picture. Many books have been written and some even recommend renting. However, you will notice they recommend investing in the stock market to multiply your money. The choice is yours. Follow your brain.

October 22, 2020

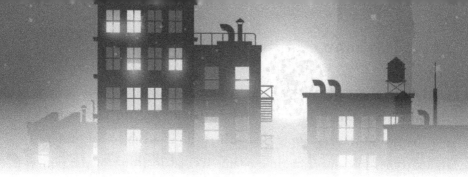

PRESIDENTIAL DEBATE

President incumbent Joe Biden is taking this pandemic seriously while the president of the United States, Donald Trump, seems to think differently. He seems to think it will just go away—even as soon as this winter. He still seems sure there will be a vaccine within a few weeks.

Of course, that would be wonderful for all of us. Many people are getting anxious or depressed with all the pressures they're under and the loss of their freedom. President Biden is more cautious and warns us to be on guard, as it will probably take longer than that—*much* longer. With the election on the horizon, he's reminding us about how long it took in the past to adapt a vaccine. Other issues have included clean water and prison reform. Donald wants more prisons, as there aren't enough people in jail, according to him.

I believe the US still has the death penalty. Pity. Joe Biden pointed out that there were many more Blacks in prison than Whites, asking for prison reform, not more people in jail and more treatments for drugs and alcohol. Also, that police departments must change.

There is also the subject of global warming. There must be sacrifices to bring about an end to global warming. We must improve our climate if we're to survive. Electric chargers, retrofit homes, AOC (not sure what that stands for)—they have a plan, but so far, they're hesitant to spend the money to make it a reality. Fracking needs to stop.

Cars must go to zero emissions. It looks like all the major countries in the world need to knuckle down and see that it happens. The statistics, not just world leaders, show that this is so. The subject of minority rights comes up time and time again. It's sad to think of the police harassment of Blacks.

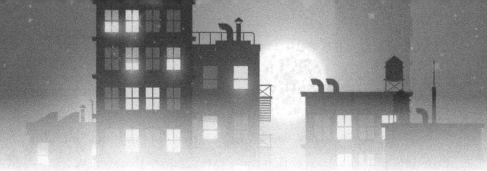

SCHOOLING - THE OLD WAY AND THE FUTURE

COVID won't last forever. We must pray for an early way out of it, but be patient. It may help to know what it was like in the past and see how we've progressed.

My middle son took a class on tin smithing, I think it was. He came home with a little shovel he had made. He also took cooking for one year. That, strangely enough, put him in good stead, as he married and had seven children and he has helped with the cooking ever since. He should have become a lawyer. His personality seemed to point that way. He chose band in high school and played the French horn. He liked acting and singing and took part in the school productions and junior orchestra. In retirement, he's enjoyed volunteering for charities, including the Red Cross.

My other son, as I recall, took extra languages. He became a linguist with about five languages under his belt. He moved to Japan and spent forty years translating from Japanese into English. He became a good scuba diver and travelled around the world every chance he got. He picks up the languages pretty well when he needs them when travelling.

My only daughter took sewing. She had a marvellous teacher and became a wonderful seamstress, making her own clothing, baby quilts, and all sorts of things. Her career took her to banking as a mortgage broker. Both helped her in real estate ownership.

In university, they went their different ways but for this dissertation, I will just mention those extra courses that were necessary in high school along with their required subjects. University may be discussed at another time but not for now.

The following trades are provided for your consideration and might apply now or once we've moved on from the days of COVID.

- Cement layer
- Bricklayer
- Carpenter
- Plumber
- Stonemason
- Elevator repairer
- Painter
- Shoe repairer
- Gardner
- Swim instructor
- Tai-chi teacher
- Gym instructor
- Auto mechanic
- Car salesman
- Craftsman (native or otherwise)
- Mineralogist
- Diamond miner (up north)
- Seamstress
- Chef
- Veterinarian

- Pet Store Owner
- Caregiver
- Librarian
- Author
- Journalist
- Beekeeper
- Book Binder
- Publisher
- Printer
- Butcher
- Baker

And the list goes on. The difference may be that because there are so many choices and school space is scarce, perhaps the students could go out into the community or experts could come into the classroom. How would you feel if Wayne Gretzky came to visit your class?

I could mention my husband, Chas. He was brought up in London, England, and he talked about this gentleman of means who used to come to the school and act as a guide and took the students to all kinds of places in the city, including art galleries, the Victoria and Albert Museum, Buckingham Palace, down the Thames to Greenwich and all sorts of historical monuments within reach. Charles tells of how much that changed his life. What would change your life that you would like to say or do when COVID ends?

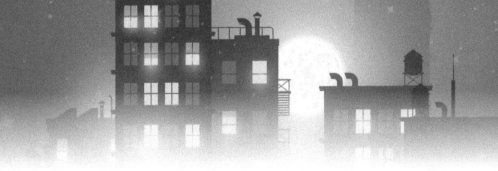

WHY KNOWING YOUR
HISTORY IS IMPORTANT

It may go back a generation or three to fly around the world to see the big picture and why you have so many more advantages, putting aside global warming and the pandemic. Grandpa Smith came from a farm in Ohio, as far as I know, and was the son of a Methodist pastor. He married my grandmother in Wisconsin. They moved around a lot. Finally, to Minnesota. My grandmother stayed home and did the household chores and raised canaries and a parrot, I believe. Grandpa Smith and their parents before them hunted for furs and skins as well as farmed but it was the natives that made the moccasins they wore and jackets for winter and beaded them both. It's funny what things stick in your mind. Grandpa raised jersey cows.

The children probably attended school until grade eight. They were needed to help on the farm, so high school was probably out of the question. The girls helped their mother.

Now, I don't know the details but the young Smiths had no children. My mother, Belle and my Aunt Minnie were raised by Alex and Jessica Smith. To my knowledge, my mother (Mabel Belle) never found out who her real parents were. Minnie's children were able to find their Scandinavian roots, but they weren't related to each other. We have school records of Minnie going to school in Duluth but nothing for Mother so far. When in Minneapolis, I found records of a girl with the same name as Mother going to secretarial school, but it was never confirmed that it was her. I don't even know if typewriters were around in 1910 or 11. Now that we have DNA records to help us, we'll never give up on finding her real parents. She told us she was born in Duluth, Minnesota, but no records have been found. We know that Alex and his brothers were horse lovers. They all immigrated to Saskatchewan in 1912 and homesteaded in the Riverhurst section of Saskatchewan by the Saskatchewan River along with son-in-law Mel Anderson and Minnie, of course, and uncle James Smith (always referred to as Doc Smith), who drove the ferry across the river. Mother married Chester William Ray in 1913 in Moose Jaw, Saskatchewan. There is no record that they were hit by the terrible typhoon that destroyed a great part of Regina. As typhoons have a habit of coming down in one place and missing another, they may have been saved, being many miles south of the city. My sister Dorothy and I never met any of those relatives.

In 1918, Grandpa Alex and Jessie, along with Mel and Minnie went back to Minnesota. Chester and Mabel Belle and their family moved to Regina, the capital of Saskatchewan. Please forgive me for rambling on. I'll leave it there. It's found in my book *Finding My Family*. If you have immigrant ancestors, I'd be glad to hear about them.

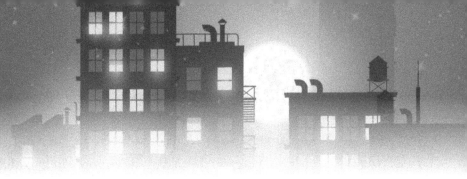

THE DIRTY THIRTIES

When I wrote that heading, my helper looked at it and had no idea what that was all about, so I'd better explain that that was the name given to the prairies North and South of America because of the huge drought that occurred. As far as I knew as a child, I had no father, grandfather, uncles, aunts, or other relatives. There was just my sister, Dorothy, and I—and our mother, who worked cleaning floors and the office of The Regina Pure Milk. I believe the pay was about fifty cents a day. That wouldn't buy you a cup of coffee today. She earned a little extra by knitting mittens and gloves for the linemen who were putting up telephone lines across Saskatchewan in the winter.

During the '30s, jobs were almost impossible to find. I mention it because there are those gurus who predict another depression as they had back then for several reasons. One is that unemployment has risen enormous amounts due to the pandemic. Another, is because of the great lack of rain in many states and provinces. They're suffering droughts from North to South. The melting of the glaciers doesn't help. People spend money as if there's no tomorrow. Also, the attitudes of banks and the stock market, which are racing ahead at magnificent speed. Huge companies are able to pay down their loans and other obligations. There are governments to contend with. They must make the right decisions, and the people must agree with those decisions to prevent the downturn ahead.

Of course, I could be wrong. I often am. I *hope* I am. One thing we know is that things won't be the same. Many things will be as different as night and day. People will make it so. Our inclination is to keep things the same, but many things are broken and must be fixed. You may not agree, but you are the future. There will be inventions indescribable right now. Things for good and things for evil. You are part of that future. I am not.

I like to consider what seniors might enjoy:

1. Seniors will each have their own private room in a wonderful care home for the duration of their life.

2. Education will be available for everybody.

3. Caregivers won't have to shuffle from one job to another, so germs and infections won't spread that way.

4. Nurses' rates and other caregivers will increase, as they've been fighting for.

5. Global warming: An effort will be made, big and small, to come in way ahead of predictions.

6. Police governance: Law enforcers will be an example of exemplary treatment of their fellow man regardless of race, colour, education, or station in life.

7. Mental health: Police officers will call for appropriate support to help when necessary to intervene.

8. Education will be provided regarding the effects of taking drugs and the consumption of alcohol.

9. Homelessness: This huge problem will no longer be; it will be eradicated.

10. Education concerning pandemics in general: Isolation, treatments, and vaccines will all be covered in the public school system.

11. Safer roads/vehicles: Citizen thoughts will be reflected upon to aid in accident prevention.

12. Tourism

13. Senior abuse, which is seldom taught or understood.

AMERICAN ELECTION DAY

Joe Biden (D) vs. Donald Trump (R)

Would it be safe to say that Donald Trump doesn't take advice? He doesn't have advisors; he has *enablers*. He claims he has won the election before all the votes are counted. The score is close for sure, but he came back with his family before the press and for days on end wouldn't agree that he hadn't been re-elected. As a Canadian, I shouldn't interfere, but I'm awfully glad that the recount at his request was found out that he was short of votes to remain the president of the United States. His opinions on COVID may have had something to do with it. Also the Black vote. I was really proud of them. I remember that my mother didn't vote. President Biden got busy right away, trying to correct some of the things that had been neglected.

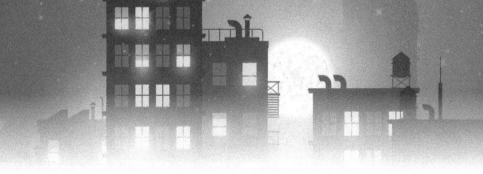

PURCHASING HOUSES

People come to me at times and ask my advice about purchasing a house. In these trying times, I hesitate to say there is a right or wrong time to buy a house but I'll say a bit about getting ready to make your purchase. Things seem to be very brisk around Vancouver this year, and prices are up 13 percent already, but no one would have guessed that would have happened. What works for one may not work for another. Everyone is different. It helps to have a healthy bank balance in the first place. If not, you need to begin living as if you were back in university, counting every penny. The government sometimes will give first-time homebuyers a boost to help them get started. We were never offered one, but we did help a grandson buy a home on those grounds. He had a good job with good pay and is paying extra each month to get it paid off.

I hope he's also buying stocks to have a portfolio to fall back on. A mortgage helper would be nice as well, and it was quite a bargain to start within an area of nice homes. His work seems to be permanent, and he's healthy. I believe it's easy to get back and forth to work. There were some repairs to be made but he's a carpenter as well.

On the other hand, I remember when my husband Bill was in the Canadian Navy, there was a young man who told me he and his wife had saved 10 percent of their pay for a house, but every year, prices went up 10 percent—not a good spot to be in. We had three children and no money, and as a last-ditch effort, we borrowed money from my father-in-law, which allowed us to buy what we called "an old junker." We managed to pay the loan back, but my mother-in-law said that her husband hadn't slept until he got his money.

There is no magic bullet. You can rent a place if it's available, but rents go up too.

Some young people built their own place, hiring trade workers to help them while they lived with their folks. This isn't so popular today. Not with so many regulations; it may be difficult.

The reason I prefer purchasing houses rather than renting? I usually fall back on the fact that when a couple comes to retirement age, that is often the one thing they have to show for their years of work. Maybe a little money in the bank or a large government cheque each month. Perhaps a company pension—perhaps not. It's hoped, of course, that they have some investments and other savings, but when COVID struck, the government surmised that everyone lived paycheque to paycheque. They also made it illegal for the landlord to give their renters notice. However, if an owner had a mortgage on the house, even if the payments were forgiven—let's say postponed—they would have to be paid eventually, and of course, the interest goes on, the light bill goes on, the gas goes on, the yearly taxes go on. Owning a house is arguably still worth it, and if you have a mortgage helper you can really count your blessings.

That's why I must say that something could go wrong with your job, or heaven forbid your marriage or your health or the health of someone in the family. I would say in the period of ninety years, there could be any number of difficulties, so you'd be wise to prepare. I could tell you some of mine but the book would be too thick. I didn't say it would be easy, but I do say it will be worth it.

Don't depend on the government if you can help it. People from the US (and I'm related to half of them) tell me I'm so lucky that Canada has free medical. I laugh to myself. To them, it looks free, but nothing is free. We pay through gas taxes and other taxes. Americans understand that when they come for a visit and have to buy gas for their car or motor home. Perhaps that's why the gasless car is so slow in getting developed. If gas prices double, maybe global warming would slow down because everyone would vie for a gasless vehicle.

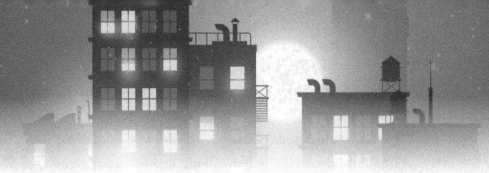

COVID, HAS THERE BEEN ANYTHING GOOD ABOUT IT?

This chapter may be a tough one. In life, even the worst calamities rarely turn out as bad as we expect. Let's hope the same holds true for COVID. Therefore, I'll have to dig and see if I can find out something good right now.

Actually, pollution went down, according to the press. Many people personally didn't feel it, but it was measurable. Millions lost their jobs. That wasn't good, but they no longer had to leave home and drive great distances to work. Therefore, they didn't have to drive, which saved money on gas and resulted in much less pollution. That was measurable.

Some were able to stay home with the children and not have to pay a sitter. There was no 9:00 or 5:00 rush, so there weren't as many car accidents either. Car insurers were giving out refunds. That would have been unimaginable before. Schools closed. This was a negative for sure but only until the teachers and powers that be figured out how the children could do their lessons online and how to modernize (maybe not the correct word) the classrooms and playgrounds so the children could continue with their education. (*Improvise* might have been a better word for changing the classrooms, but I leave it deliberately.) It was discovered that very few children got COVID, but it was best to err on the side of caution. We should be thankful for that and put it on the plus side. Another plus: the mothers and caregivers didn't have to take children to school.

Television stations didn't have to ask their guests to come into the station. This saved visitors from flying in from Timbuktu. The audiences at home and elsewhere could watch as they talked, sang, or performed wherever they preferred, even from their own home living rooms.

The elderly had to stay home—that's true and that had its disadvantages. They were at the most risk of dying of COVID, so going out or having anyone come in was risky. However, many services appeared to bring in meals and groceries being discouraged from going out to the shops or wherever else there could be crowds.

Those who lived with their family were allowed to remain in what they called a "bubble." Some of us are alone but nonetheless thankful for our friends. We have to count our pennies for extra services, but the telephone, TV, and computer have been great company even if we can't get out to visit.

Getting to the bank is difficult. Even mailing a letter poses problems. Getting a doctor's appointment may be difficult, and medical care in the hospital will have to wait. However, Handy Dart is available to most as long as you wear a mask. It can help you get to appointments.

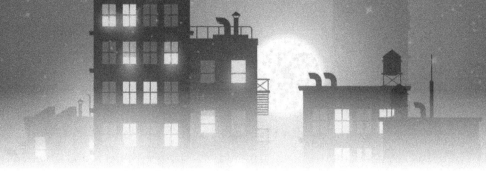

DISADVANTAGES

Swimming pools, beaches, gymnasiums, libraries, restaurants, bakeries, coffee shops, offices, and small owner shops were all closed down or had certain restrictions. The government did its best, but many companies went out of business entirely. Mental breakdowns turned quiet neighbours into Halloween freakshows, with people blaming everything except themselves for conditions they couldn't control. Some blamed people who looked different than them or who came from a different country for all their troubles and the world's troubles. Police turned from "that kind befriender on the corner" to a tyrant with a gun and boots strong enough to do lethal damage. People in the United States took to marching in the streets to voice their distress, but some armed themselves with weapons of destruction aimed at breaking windows and yes, protecting themselves from the very men who were supposedly there to protect them.

I remember years ago when teenagers here in Vancouver went wild after a hockey game. I don't know what the motive was, but apparently, the wrong team won. They took to the downtown streets, smashing glass, bouncing on cars and just wreaking havoc on Granville Street and passed the Bay. The police moved in, but then the attention went to protecting themselves from the cops or what they said. Many young people were hauled away to the police station and given police records that would stay with them all their lives for destroying other people's property. Parents were called, and I know some were taken to court, fined and maybe, served jail time.

Pictures turned up in the paper the next day, and parents who didn't even dream their child could do such a thing found them absolutely out of control. These kids who worshipped that great hockey player Wayne Gretzky had certainly let the team down. He had the motto to 1. Prepare. 2. Work hard. 3. Motivate yourself. 4. Have a desire to improve. 5. Create an environment to make it happen, on and off the ice. *What were these guys thinking?* I wondered. May it never be repeated.

VIRTUAL TELEVISION

What would we do without virtual vision during COVID? I couldn't say, but I'd like to think that it's right on time for the public to embrace it. The technology was already there.

We can now go to church by connecting to the Internet without contacting anyone except our immediate family at our elbow. We're on *Zoom*! We can see the Tabernacle Choir in Salt Lake City singing hymns to all the world with the orchestra, which we could never have in our ward here in Vancouver, then become connected with the leadership just three miles away. They haven't got the mechanics of broadcasting to perfection, but every week, they improve, and every week, the numbers watching grow and grow. Someone is assigned the opening prayer; another two members give the most wonderful spiritual talks. The announcements are given by the bishopric. Then, someone else gives the closing prayer, and again the choir sings another beloved hymn. It's going to be difficult to go back to normal when we have to turn up every Sunday morning at the meeting house and be there in person. However, it will be wonderful to meet with our friends again in person and testify our belief in our Savior and the truth of the gospel. "President Nelson, you're such a blessing to all of us." Everything is possible.

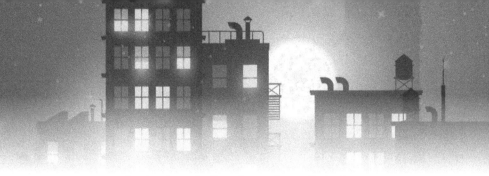

HOBBIES AND OLD-FASHIONED SKILLS

Things that you or your family might be doing or could do can be very important during COVID when you may have time dragging. You'll need to keep your brain active especially as you get older. It's best to be prepared—and active.

You'll be fortunate if you're able to keep doing the things you appreciate during COVID. You may be under a great deal of pressure, facing shortened or lengthened hours, or even the threat of losing your job—or other circumstances in your family when sickness prevails.

I don't know your hobbies, so take time to write them down, and you'll be able to come back to add if something crosses your mind. The following are just those of my present and past. Yours could be far different.

My mother taught me to do spool knitting before I went to kindergarten. She was an excellent knitter, and besides knitting for my sister and I, sometimes knit gloves for money when things were tough. Actually, times were *always* tough.

I had my first lemonade stand when I was ten. My girlfriend and I sold on the street corner to the Air Force members returning to the barracks. Sometimes, they gave us a nickel for our efforts. That enterprise lasted a few days. I think her mother ran out of lemons.

In high school, I set pins at a bowling alley to make spending money. It was a good job, but perhaps my school work suffered.

I learned to type at business college and Balfour Tech. Well rewarded. Now five-year-olds know more about computers than I do, I'm sure.

I also chopped wood. It takes certain skills, but it kept the home fires burning.

Then, I did bookkeeping. Everyone should learn this. I worked for the Anglican College while going to university. They were kind, but I was poor at my debits and credits. Mr. Bell Irving was my boss.

Next, I painted greenware. I hardly recognized my work when it came out of the kiln.

While in school, I made artwork with HB pencils. Okay, but the teacher kept my only masterpiece.

I looked after two old maids and their mother while attending business classes. My teacher recommended I quit, but she didn't know that was the only money I had to buy my mother a birthday present.

Later, I made ice-cream cones at Regina Beach. That ice cream was frozen so hard, I couldn't get it out of the tub and into the cone. The owner gave up on me. I was glad.

I helped a new mother with her twins. The house was spotless already.

Washing dishes at the Wascana ice cream store wasn't particularly exciting. I quit before they invented dishwashers.

I recommend that every child works for McDonald's as early as they'll take you. Their training is excellent. Most of all, they teach you how to interact with people. They do have one problem. They're inclined to give you more hours than you should take when you're attending high school, and the pay isn't enough to stay there very long. Move on.

Learn to cook by yourself. Invent something everyone will like. Make your own recipe book. Personalize.

You should also complete high school. Get the highest marks you can. (Yes, that does require studying—a *lot* of studying). I'll admit that I don't even spell well. I didn't complete high school, but I did get my junior matriculation. I started earning wages full-time. There were no jobs in Regina, so at a friend's urging, I moved to Toronto. I also finally attended business school. The teacher even changed my handwriting forever. Miss Treen was such a darling.

I still can't spell. Spellcheck was made especially for me.

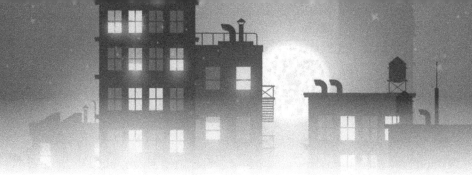

PRESENT DAYS DURING THE PANDEMIC

"D on't ever be too busy to stop and appreciate everything in your life. Success without fulfilment will lead to your ultimate downfall, so always take time to appreciate the life you have." (Author unknown)

This is a glimpse of my life in a hundred-year-old house.

I have an elevator of sorts to allow me to get into my back door. It's rather new, but frankly, it's called the lift that won't lift. I called in an elevator specialist to fix it, as I couldn't carry my groceries up the stairs or my walker down them. He told me he would fix it, but the charge would be $500.00 for one hour. If he had known how much of my pension that was, he should have turned me down, but I thought if he fixed it, the cost would be worth it.

However, it only worked for a short while, and I had to get someone else to fix it. The original installers had long since gone out of business. Another workman appeared, and the price was lower, but it didn't work for long, and he had to come back. Again, he repaired it and said he would be back with a part. It did work for a month or two, but I was fed up. I left it as it was and took the stairs with help. Finally, my son came from Alberta and he tried to fix it. No luck. He phoned for help and they tried but couldn't get the thing in order. The latest is that he phoned an elevator company and everything is on hold, as I haven't heard from them and worry about what their charges would be and whether or not they'd be any good.

I put in a new heating system a year before COVID came along. People ask what it cost and then gasp when I tell them, but I'm happy the savings over time will atone for the price. The father of the company was in my writing group in Delta years ago.

The roof. It's apparent that it needs doing. It will cost more than the house cost years ago.

The garden. My grown grandson lives downstairs and looks after the lawn in the summer and shovels the snow in the winter in exchange for cheap rent. Not a bad deal. We have to have trimmers in for the hedge, which must be at least seventy-five years old.

Painters came over to the house and painted the old trim purple. I asked for dark charcoal, but that's the way it turned out. Purple isn't my favourite colour, and the blue they put on for charcoal would never pass the scrutiny of my father-in-law, James Hogg, a professional house painter. He taught me that blue fades, so the professionals avoid it at all costs. I had the trim repainted.

Even having it redone didn't help. Ah well.

Partly because of the trees, the concrete sidewalks in front of the house and down the street need work. They're as wavy as the Atlantic Ocean with cracks upon cracks. The city will do them in due time when the repair crew gets around to it.

My bricklayer husband was skilled in fixing electric items around the house. He learned at night school. I am gradually moving up to LED lights to save on the electric bill.

The drapes and windows will have to wait as well. I could lower the temperature a bit in summer and heighten it in winter with the right technology. Fans are my main summer cooling. I must say that they are not likely energy-saving, but I try not to waste. Actually, Vancouver isn't into air conditioning, but that may change in the future with global warming.

There is a great deal of talk about gasless cars. In 2019, the price of gas is down but what goes down can also go up. It's not about price; it's about conservation. Also, there is talk of extending the sky train out to Langley, thirty miles farther east than the present lines go and out west to the University of British Columbia. Yes, that will help, but governments usually drag their feet. They could switch the tables on us all, and why not take the university out to the country? No one is anxious to do that, but a few years ago, I helped raise money for Fraser Valley University along with the owner and family of a popular family in Delta near Vancouver. I was so happy to be of a little help. I kept thinking of how wonderful it would be if Delta had what we call "post-education" and the grandchildren wouldn't have to go all the way to Vancouver to receive higher education. Well, the joke was on me. The Fraser Valley University was built many miles up north in Prince George. Our loss was their gain. Delta still doesn't have a university, but looking back, I'm very happy how it turned out, as my daughter-in-law and many thousands of others got their degrees up north where it was really needed. She became an excellent nurse.

A good bus service is also heralded. Every trip taken on the bus is a car left at home. During COVID, bus transportation is lessened mainly because schools and businesses are shut down. Masks must be worn and stops have lengthened, which affects me, but I haven't gone out much since COVID.

We can't wait for governments or industries to manifest everything to save the problem; we each must do our part.

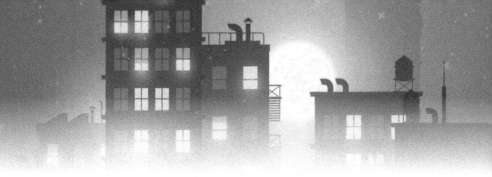

PAST SAD EVENTS

Although Canada and its close neighbours spell a few words differently, many here have US roots and associations. When our neighbours grieve, we grieve. I still remember the day President Kennedy was shot by Lee Harvey Oswald. Jackie Kennedy was saved by a whisker, as they say. I've always been thankful for that, and I can still see in my mind his two small children at the funeral. It was beyond sad. The crime has never been solved. You always remember the day of tragedies. I remember missing a dental appointment that day with eyes glued to the screen. I'm Scottish by infusion if not by blood (I don't know who my father was) and was shocked when that dentist charged me just the same.

We don't observe the day of 9/11, but most of us can remember exactly when it happened. In Vancouver, it came on the news early in the morning. I was fast asleep when my husband came in and said, "Put on the TV! Something terrible is happening!" Not knowing what to expect, I turned it on.

At first, I thought I was looking at some science fiction film, and all I wanted to do was go back to sleep, but then I turned the station. The same thing was on that channel as well. I couldn't believe it, but they were repeating it over and over. When I realized what was happening, it was really unbelievable! Two planes crashing into the high rises of New York City! It couldn't be! Who would do a thing like that? The news was intimating that more planes were heading to Washington and the Pentagon building. Later in the day, they said they even had Seattle as a target. The bad news got worse and worse. Thousands of people were plunging to their deaths. The high-rises were crumbling to the ground before our eyes, and it was all being broadcast around the world. It became known as 911. It will go down in history as one of the most terrible days in American history.

I was to hear later that my sister Helen had been up in Canada visiting at that time, but as soon as she heard the news, she had her husband turn the car around and head back to Seattle in spite of the fact that Seattle was number five on the list to bomb. My niece was also in Canada, and she, too, shortened her holiday and headed back to Seattle.

I can even remember even the first day of World War II. We were in Vancouver—my mother, my sister, and I—and people started putting dark curtains on the windows. I was ten years old. I remember the men signing up for the Army and showing up in their uniforms. They said it was the first time in their lives that they got a good pair of boots. Little did they know what was ahead of them. They were off to save their country, and they did but not without great sacrifice.

I tell all this because we will all remember COVID. We write about it, and we want others to do the same. To die of COVID-19 is not a pretty sight. Our words together may make a difference. It will become a part of history, and we need to remember and not have to repeat it.

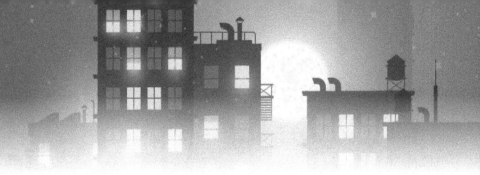

FINANCIAL HEALTH

A s I may have said before, over the course of the next few months, take a good look at your financial health. If you did it once, do it again. Nine months have gone by since COVID started. Did you think it would be like this? Did you think it would be as long as this?

Did you think the government would step in and pay the first month's rent? I figured they presumed everyone lived hand to mouth. Of course, they could have been right.

Or did they think they would have a panic on their hands of thousands and thousands of people?

They already had thousands of homeless that they were unable to tackle.

Perhaps they weren't so worried about the owners and how they would pay their lines of credit or mortgage. I held my breath, as I owe both. My tenants lost their jobs but all paid their rents.

If I'm not able to pay my line of credit I would have to sell my stock—probably at the wrong time. My Riffs & RRSPs are long gone because of my age. I had little in the bank.

I depended on my rentals almost entirely. However, I've been blessed.

The best thing that could happen was for the banks to lower their interest rates for everyone.

They always paid little for your money, but the rate charged had gone up—although historically speaking, it wasn't so high.

Lines of credit had crept up substantially. Now was the time to take action.

So many companies were shutting down or forced to close due to contamination. No one wanted this virus to take over.

The government encouraged us all to hunker down and protect ourselves, but at the same time to help the restaurants and businesses however possible.

I decided it was the wrong time to spend money beyond necessity. I had just taken a course on self-reliance and had managed to try unsuccessfully to live without a visa.

My pension is low, but by buying nothing but the essentials, I could do it—not shopping for new clothes, eating out, or ordering in.

Without anything unforeseen, I'll reach my goal. Sooner is better than later

I got into a habit lately of making automatic payments through the bank of all these things I can.

Each month, I can go over my regular account if I have to.

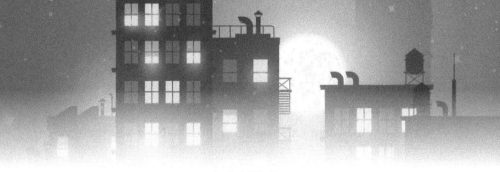

ANTS

What have itty-bitty ants got to do with the COVID pandemic? Well, let's just say we need a little humour to keep going. The ants helped me do just that.

What they are doing around the house in November is what I want them to tell me. I'll bet you wouldn't find them in Saskatchewan at this time of year.

I first noticed them in the bathroom marching up and down in the crevices of the tiles on the floor, which I had taken for clean. Soon, their brothers and sisters came in about noon, and they all headed for a smooth sector where there must have been something edible. I've heard in the past that ants were going to be the last creatures on earth as they are the cleaner-uppers, cleaner than any cleaning lady. As I watched these itsy-bitsy busy creatures, they seemed so organized, so aware of what they were doing, so wanting all their relatives in the nest someplace to receive the bounty of their efforts that I couldn't bear to crush them under my slippery feet. This pandemic had changed me. I thought deeply and noted that these little black specs should have the privilege of living and that I should help them to outlive mankind, which seemed to be getting ill and dying at record numbers. I sang softly to myself as I gingerly left the room.

As the afternoon wore on, it seemed to be getting dark about 3:00. I returned to the bathroom. The ants seemed to have disappeared.

No such luck. I entered the kitchen, and they were bustling on the stove of all places beside some left-over food. They hardly hesitated as they looked up at me as if to say, "Just doing our job."

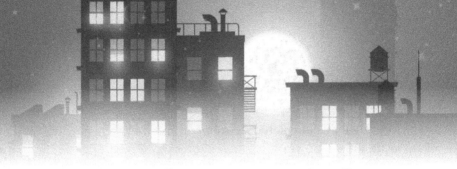

BEING SELF RELIANT
DURING COVID-19

We all seem to blame high taxes on the government. Believe it or not, though, there are countries with higher taxes than Canada, and they seem to be doing all right. Ask the Norwegians, the Brits or whomever you please, but they seem to cope.

The answer seems to be self-reliance. Try not to depend on the government. There are courses out there to help you but, in the meantime, maybe these thoughts may help you cope.

1. This one may be quite a challenge, but it's worth pondering the benefits. Pay tithes and offerings. I do. It's tough, but I need all the divine help I can get, and I admire all those who do also.

2. Managing money is a learning experience. I wasn't always good with money, but I can say I have improved a little. Remember that it's not learned in school unless things have changed a great deal. When I got to the third year at UBC, I chose a subject that was about investing, but remember: the course didn't choose me.

3. I do have a Visa card, but everyone should beware of the pitfalls. You pay for it. One way or another, the bank seems to

get paid. Either they charge you indirectly or they charge the merchant so he has to up the price to pay his charges so you'll pay for it, but if you don't pay it in full each month, the interest is enough to put the kids through college. Need I say more? You'll probably spend more than if you had to come up with the cash.

4. I put down, "Be careful who your friends and acquaintances are. You can't choose your relatives."

5. Remember that it seems like every month has its own emergencies. Yours may be different than mine, more or less, but make a list if you disagree, and you'll be surprised or fortunate: COVID may make things different. You should be on top of things to get through this unscathed.

6. Have money set aside. The government of Canada figured people spent all their paycheque every week, so they gave everyone a week's pay. Those that were in that situation and facing the pandemic (in all innocence, of course) would be close to losing their jobs or losing their business (not as quickly, mind you), losing their life because of the pandemic, or losing a member of their family. Millions died of the Spanish flu. Many lives were lost from SARS. We just don't know how many. We can do all that is asked of us, but there are no guarantees. It may take longer than you can imagine to get things under control and get businesses started up again. No one knows. With the latest technology at our fingertips, we have a great advantage, but the prognosis isn't certain. A year? Longer? It's necessary to

find an inoculation that will work; then, it needs to be given to everyone in the world because as long as it's contagious, it will be passed on. It will help to be separated from each other, but that's difficult—more difficult in some areas than others.

7. Get a good accounting system. Find out why some people pay less income tax than others. Then, change your life if necessary. Don't just sit back and complain. Save as if you might be laid off. Mother used to say "Save for a rainy day." We had many of those. Get rid of debts. Imagine what it would be like if there were a forest fire, a tornado, a flood, another war, or heaven forbid, a drought that lasted ten years like it did in the '30s. Read your history. You'll learn more than you ever dreamed was possible. Take courses. You might have to get help from family members or business associates—or, more likely, people close to you may need your help. Give the money you can but as a gift. Don't expect it back. Many a friendship has been seared by expecting it back. There will be another pandemic, sorry to say. We don't know when. Let's hope nothing like this will happen again. Sorry to have said that, but be prepared just in case.

8. Family obligations, too, must be considered. You may or may not be the main breadwinner, but it's imperative that the whole family works together in harmony. Decide on what's most important and how much must go into that account. Also, consider how much you'll have to put away and at what interval so it won't seem like so much when it's weekly or monthly. My mother had a saying which was widely known.

"Good, better, best, never let it rest, until the good is better and the better best."

9. Help a charity. You might ask, "How can my giving money to a charity help me?" I'm inclined to say "It just does." Many of you who are already giving to your favourite charity would probably agree and write me at my email, Curdsandray2002@ Yahoo.ca (making us both happy). I would be glad to hear from you. I would think that we are kindred spirits, but I think you would also like to hear of my experiences, and I hear unkind things about charities which you will never hear from me. First of all, you have to decide how much you can contribute. Let's start with "nothing." I want you to be able to feel good about what you feel you can't do. Therefore, what you may be able to do if you can't afford any money is contribute time.

    My one son volunteers at a hospital. He has no medical background, and I don't know what he does there, but I feel they are very glad to have him. He is retired (shows you how old I am) and used to go from Lethbridge to a town down the line twice a week and bring a load of necessities for the Red Cross back to the city. Nowadays he can't do that because he can't drive because of his eyesight, but he still wants to help. My other son helped with the Salvation Army in Abbotsford, British Columbia. What he did I do not know, and if he's still helping, I do not know. I used to help with the food bank's collections twice a year, and I found that enjoyable. I worked for the Red Cross when I was seven. It probably set me up for life. I only stuffed envelopes and put on stamps. Nowadays, I have many letters asking for financial help. There are over nine thousand charities in Canada, and they all seem to know my address. I can't help them all, but I do have to try and please as many as possible. Three, in particular, are dear to my heart, and they know who I am, but there are others I want to show that I admire for the work they are doing, and personally, I like to send $20.00 or more. Nevertheless, with less, I don't get the income tax advantage, and without that, I can't give as much. However, even with $5.00 from each person, if 5 million people did that alone it would be $25,000,000, and they would say, "Thank you very much." Some pay the postage. Some do not. The lady at the post office knows me well and knows I pick out the prettiest stamps or those most appropriate. I am quite fussy. I don't know my postman, but every day, he brings me more requests.

I'll have to admit that donations to local hospitals where the family and I have ended up and may in the future are common; naturally, I want the best equipment and the best services. I remember my husband, Charlie being in the Delta Hospital. When he got out, I decided we should show our appreciation—especially as they needed money to build an extension with new technology included. We became members of the Delta Hospital Foundation. I thought nothing more of it until one Sunday at church, a member stopped me to say he had seen our name in the local newspaper. I gasped as it was rather a big donation for us but a small donation in the big scheme of things. I looked it up in the paper, and there it was close to our neighbour who gave a million dollars. Actually, people like us and our neighbours do things like that to be a secret for obvious reasons.

I've heard people say that rich people give money just to get their names in the paper. I know how untrue that is and this is why. They give the money and the hospital puts their name on the extension or whatever. For that reason, I will not mention the many hospitals, wards, nurseries, and old folks' homes that have been built by people everywhere. I'm sure they don't do it with popularity in mind. I cringe when onlookers make remarks like that or even think it. Their donations may have saved my life. Yes, I know what it's like to sleep in the hallway of a hospital and to be kicked out of a bed or two to make room for someone who needed the bed more than I did. My efforts are small in comparison, but I'm still here on Earth, so something is working. Now, what does this have to do with getting your finances in order? Some would say "Everything" because if you have the welfare of others as you get your own house in order, you'll be happier, have more reason to live, realize the meaning of life, and accomplish those things you are trying to achieve, COVID or no COVID.

10. Save money on stamps. Sending many small donations at $1.00 approximately per stamp can really add up. I like the donations which include the postage, even if they say, "Use your own stamp and it will mean a greater donation for us." That is correct, but I don't do that because, number one, they get a discount on the stamps I'm sure, and they only do that because they're more likely to get a donation from someone

who doesn't have to go out and buy a stamp to mail it. I love the lady at our post office, and she agreed with me when I wrote a letter to the post office general and told him that the stamps nowadays were a disgrace. I used the word *crummy*. I suppose I shouldn't have, but he never got the letter. In the old days, it used to be free to send the postmaster general but apparently not now. Would you believe that the letter came back? I had sent in my opinion on how terrible the stamps were and suggested they consider Naval stamps and cartoons on the seven-book series I had written on the Royal Canadian Naval history from 1945–1954 when my husband, William Ronald Hogg, was in the forces. I also complained about buying a child's game I had bought at the dollar store for $4.00. The postage was $16.00. Stamps on the package: none, absolutely zero. There was a time when you could use stamps or have a sticker put on the parcel. That, too, seems to have gone by the wayside. I don't think children even save stamps now, with email being so convenient.

11. But I digress. I have a stamp collection that goes back to 1946 when I worked in the Simpson's warehouse in Toronto. I collected all kinds of beautiful stamps that really meant something and were sometimes works of art.

Back to helping others. I'm amazed by how much even young children have given to charity through their own efforts. The lemonade stands are still around, perhaps, but they're so much more creative than we were when we were young. They have earned thousands of dollars, one at a time, for healthcare workers and all sorts of causes during this first

COVID year. They are so much smarter than my girlfriend and I were during the second world war with our lemonade stand to earn money for the Red Cross and the airmen stopping by and giving us money even if they didn't particularly want to drink the lemonade. I remember our venture only lasted as long as the friend's mother's lemons lasted.

12. Another thing that amazed me this year was Americans actually wearing poppies. Congratulations! We were brought up with the poem in our heart, "In the fields, the poppies grow, between the crosses row on row," commemorating the soldiers lost in World War I. "That mark the place and in the sky . . ." We would buy a poppy for Remembrance Day, November 11, 1918, at 11 a.m. ". . . the larks still singing, fly. The price per poppy was little, but that money helped the veterans.

13. Car insurance. In British Columbia, car insurance is looked after by the provincial insurance called ICBC. There are many people who want that changed to private companies because they think it would be cheaper. Instead, maybe if there would be fewer careless drivers, the rates would go down. In fact, with COVID, everyone got a refund due to the fact there were fewer cars on the road and fewer accidents.

14. Acquire insurance on your home. You can't learn too much, but you're always insured even if you don't know it. I'm half-joking because even when you haven't insured your possessions, I tell people that they are insured. I call it "self-insurance." In other words, you, yourself, are the insurer.

I can also say that you can insure anything. I didn't say how difficult it might be. Insurance companies, in my opinion, hate to part with money. Therefore, when they insure your home, apartment, or anything else, I found out the hard way that when water came down from the upstairs suite through our suite, "Oh we don't insure water damage." Woe was me. I paid for all the repairs and cancelled with that company. Shortly afterwards, in our house on inspection, the insurance company insisted that we replace the hot water tank. Our plumber insisted that it didn't need replacing. Therefore, the insurer cancelled the policy. I finally gave in, replacing the complete heating system at a cost of $21,000.00. When that happened, I could no longer afford the insurance. Life insurance was also complicated. On a seaman's earnings, it was difficult to buy insurance. However, Bill's insurance man was a friend of the family and suggested a life insurance policy so small that, looking back, it was more or less useless. When time went by, another insurance approached him and sold him a $5,000.00 policy, which, when he died, was a little help, but for some reason, only one-half of the policy went to me and the rest was held until the children were grown. Figure that one out. It's often said that insurance salesmen are inclined to sell the policies that they make the most money on. In the time of a pandemic, I do think everyone should have some kind of insurance, especially if they have a family. The Navy did eventually have insurance available to the men, but that was after my time. The pension died with the sailor. It was called the old pension plan. Much later they did get a new pension plan but it was too late for our family. You need the largest pension you can build in these days of inflation—especially with COVID still in the picture. Buy the largest amounts you can for the cheapest amounts of money I would say. Ask if it's pure insurance. You don't need a savings plan included.

Apartment insurance is also key. When you buy an apartment, if it's a new building, the assessments you have to pay are relatively inexpensive, as everything is practically brand new. However, you can count on those assessments to increase every year, and they can be extensive. Some buildings do accumulate a slush fund, so if you buy an apartment, you might like to check that out. Some people sell when they know costly expenses are coming along in a year or two, which will strain the budget. Disability insurance is a grand thing to have—at least on the surface and especially if your employer is paying for it. The problem comes because it is usually only in place from 9 to 5 or should we say during working hours in case you're hurt at work. If you go out after hours and get hurt—say on the football pitch—you're not covered. Also, it often has time restrictions. My granddaughter is a teacher in a city close to here. She was injured twice, both times at school which was fortunate in a way. Both injuries were the result of falls, one on the slippery coat-room floor. Both were serious and she sustained a brain injury. She was insured by the school board for five years, but regardless of her health, it ran out after that time.

I tell you this to warn you to prepare. Have some money invested. Those student loans aren't as easy to pay back as they seem, so there are two things that I suggest. If at all possible and plausible, stay home with your parents during your first two years or more of college. Have a part-time job even before you start college. Work during the summer if you possibly can. Get a bursary if possible. I remember going to UBC when the children were small. I had no choice really. There weren't student loans as there are today. Yes, it was tough. We were fortunate that we could stay with the in-laws.

Having said all that, if you have to borrow and you have no student loan to fall back on, borrow as little as you have to, but remember that your degree will be worth it. I didn't get a degree.

An idea I thought of when the children were going to college was to buy a small apartment in Spokane, Washington, I think it was. Two of my sisters and their husbands bought that bit of real estate for them to live on while they attended college away from home in Seattle. Eventually, after graduation, they either rented it out or sold it. It turned out to be a good investment.

Another good idea, though it isn't always possible, is to get a job while in college. Many students work at our local grocery store and pharmacy to earn college money. Even a small amount can make a difference to a student's lifestyle.

I haven't added anything sensational, but I'd be glad to hear about your own ideas. They say thousands of scholarships aren't picked up every year. I miraculously got a bursary in my second year.

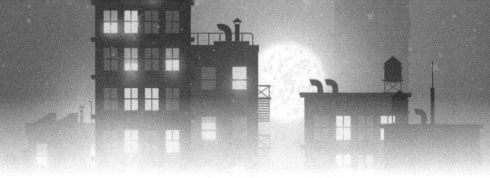

YOUR EMERGENCY
FUND REVISITED

Write down how much your emergency fund has in it or money you could get for it if you needed to cash in on short notice. The following questions will prove useful in preparing and managing your finances.

1. How long will it last?

2. What could it pay off to prevent further erosion?

3. Who could you go to for help? How much could they help you with? How much would they likely be willing to give you? Those two questions are really quite different.

4. Can you quickly put aside a one-month emergency fund? Do you think COVID-19 will end soon?

5. Could you hazard a guess when it will end? I don't like to go here, but I would say, "When we get a vaccine, what percentage will get the shots?"

6. I think of the flu shots, which we get every year, seem to be coming in late this year. Will more people line up?

7. After we do get the shots, will the recovery be swift?

PRESIDENTIAL ELECTION
USA

Actually, the world will be different starting today. The US Election count is over officially today. President Biden will make his first speech tonight at 6 p.m. Mountain Standard Time. Of course, now President Donald Trump announced that he was the new president a couple of nights ago at a quarter to midnight (three in the morning Eastern Standard Time.) I don't know why they didn't just close down at midnight and stop counting until morning. They knew what he was going to do, prone as he is to stirring the kettle.

This notable date is November 7, 2020. The result was close in some cases. We Canadians don't know why they do things in such old-fashioned ways, but President Donald Trump wanted them to just stop the counting and name him re-elected. Interesting!!! Those who didn't get their vote counted would really be up in the air. I guess President Trump would say then that he was just fooling, but he was serious; believe me.

It was too close for comfort for Biden as it was, but it was the greatest number to vote in history. Would it have been any different had the COVID pandemic not been here? It will be read and reread over the eons. It's certain that if Donald Trump had been voted in for a second session, Canada would be unhappy, although many of us don't pay attention to world politics.

127

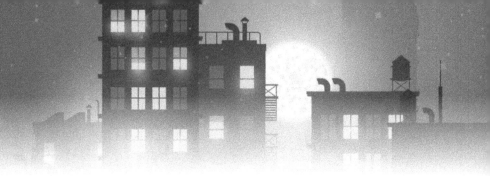

MESSAGE FROM MY SPACE HERO
CHRIS HATFIELD

Chris Hatfield, our neighbour from Victoria, just gave us a message from space. We are so fortunate to have a neighbour in space to look down at the world and see us as we really are. It's hard to believe but he called the world to let us know he'd gotten the message. I guess if Donald Trump got involved in that, he'd probably have his lawyers argue that it would be easier for them to do that than for the elect to count a few million ballots. Chris made it sound so easy to live high in the sky with knowledge, not fear, with eagerness, not trepidation. Love that guy!

If he were here today and telling me of the day, he told his wife about being chosen for such an expedition I would have to tell them of my trip from Kelowna, British Columbia, to Vancouver, British Columbia. I know he likes a laugh and a happy story. I must share it with you.

It was a long time ago—maybe before Chris was born—when I was up at Vernon, British Columbia. This is my airplane story: I was visiting my daughter Glenna; her husband, Paul; and their young children (in order from top to bottom, Abe, Andrew, and Leah). People tease me for having three grandchildren all with biblical names—the pride of my life. That weekend, I had left my bricklayer husband behind on a job on Vancouver Island, but it was time for me to get back home to Vancouver.

I wanted to look my best for my husband when I got there, so I had my hair cut and permed and—something I had always wanted to do—my ears pierced. I was tired of wearing earrings that hurt my ears and were wont to fall off and get lost. I was taking a chance but, as the saying goes: "Vanity—her name is Woman."

A short stop into Woolworth's Store for "knock 'em dead" earrings completed the ensemble. A new outfit would have to wait for the August sales. "What will Charlie say?" Such extravagance!

Paul, my son-in-law, drove me to Kelowna Airport, about an hour south of Vernon where they lived. It was a lovely day, and I felt great and anxious to get back to my husband.

Their airport was small, nestled in the Okanagan Valley, not visible from the upper atmosphere. I wouldn't be surprised if Chris, peering down from space, could see the smoke and breathe a sigh when he thought of his beloved Earth, but the forest fires they had had in the area that summer certainly could be visible as far as the eye could see. They were still smouldering up on top of the hills to the east but the worst was over—we hoped forever. I'm sure they showed from outer space.

Before long, our plane arrived with finesse, demonstrating a perfect landing on the freeway, unloading its visitors on the beautiful playground of the Okanagan Valley. I thought of my sister Ethel and her husband, Adrian, who also lived in Okanagan Valley in Washington State, although they spelled it slightly differently. I wondered that day if planes ever got lost and landed at the wrong airport. I mingled with the passengers heading toward our plane, which seemed much smaller than any plane I had been on. My throat kind of went "gulp." I was comparing it with the 747s I had flown to Europe on and beyond. "Maybe I should have taken the bus," I told myself.

"Don't be such a scaredy-cat. You know that there are no direct bus lines. You'd have to take the long route through Kamloops and the Fraser Valley. The plane will go up and come back down in a few minutes," I told myself.

Still, I had trepidations. It wasn't as if I hadn't flown before. I thought of that trip to Britain when Charlie and I celebrated our eighteenth anniversary. We had left in the beginning of December on that huge jet that flew by way of Toronto. (They didn't fly over the pole in those days—or at least not that I know of.)

We were downed in Toronto for six hours in their gigantic airport. Being the Greenhorns that we were, we eyed the passengers who could be seen devouring delectable suppers followed by the first Baked Alaskas we had ever seen. By the time we got into line, we could have eaten the flames on that delicious dessert. Alas, by then, they were all out of food. Yes, and another eight hours once we got on board.

Now, years later, standing in that line in Kamloops, they were too small to have a restaurant because of the shortness of all flights, I guessed. However, as the wind was blowing across the runway the smallness of the wings on that plane gave me the shivers. Suddenly, a tall man in line, singing happily to himself, inwardly waving to the world (I could tell), suddenly caught my ear. "Off to Vancouver?" he chirped, knowing the answer. After all, that's the only place the plane went. I remarked how happy he sounded, and he replied by telling me how glad he was to be flying that morning, and I learned he had been in Her Majesties air force and how happy that made him to be in the air again. He didn't seem nervous at all, and his chatter about his sojourn in the Naval Air Force was the happiest time of his life and his happy humming made me feel calm. "Should be a good flight." He almost sang the words. His voice seemed to be whistling down below like a herdsman in the Lake Country.

Onboard, I found it was open seating, and he'd found the seat just across from me. I'm sure he would have liked to talk to the pilot if he could. The takeoff was a bit rough, but his voice was calming, and he was pointing out the vastness of the fire—the miracle that no one had been caught by the extent of the flames. He seemed to know every landmark between us and Mother Earth. The scenery was lovely, and before we knew it, we had landed safely home.

I almost forgot the reception I got when we arrived. My husband seemed happy to see me and gave me a husbandly welcome and a word or two such as, "You got your hair done, I see." but not a word about what I had feared. He never mentioned the pierced ears.

And here it is, November, and okay to bring out and play the Christmas music. Santa is busy up north. I'd like to say COVID is forgotten, but that isn't the case. Those over sixty are still in the high-risk group. I wanted to go to the bank and the dollar store but thought better of it. Dr. Bonny Henry wants no groups except small family members. The number of people infected is increasing, but I've heard that the US may be called "dangerously high." Of course, people down there don't seem to like rules.

November 8, 2020

Who would have dreamed I would have lived this long? You think perhaps I'm going to step in and give you a lecture on how to live a long life. Actually, I can't imagine why I lived this long. Thanks to God, I guess. Maybe it was to write this book. I had a friend, Kay Charter who lived to be 105—smart as a tack, at home with her daughter (outlived her son-in-law) on Vancouver Island, so be prepared. Live right; live for others.

November 9, 2020

The US election ballots are officially counted, but ex-President Trump may still take someone to court because he didn't win. There weren't any misdeeds or miscounts, but he may have to have his say. If I have to give my opinion on why the vote was so close, I would have to say "Biden gained votes because Donald Trump's antics were so outrageous, although I have met many Americans who, in a sense, think like him. They say when asked why they don't believe in government medical insurance, "You wouldn't want me to pay for the medical expenses of everybody else in the neighbourhood, would you?" They just don't get the big picture. Pity! Many thought it was better that a sick person pays his own hospital expenses even if it cost him his home. Others think like Trump—that they shouldn't have to wear a mask or stay in small groups because COVID-19 would disappear on its own. Of course, it hasn't. It just got worse because of that "Don't tell me what to do attitude." It still exists. Some people never learn.

That's also why so many people have guns in the US. They use them getting away with murder or manslaughter—from the police down. No London Bobbies there. Please tell me I'm wrong.

Taxes on imports. The US pays taxes on Canadian metals. Canada then has to pay taxes on US metals. This was changed by a Mexico, US, and Canada agreement, but Trump renegotiated the NATO agreement during his first four years. Obviously popular by some, not by others. Idaho pig farmers wanted taxes on bacon from Canada. The list went on and on. Then, they wanted it on cheese, oil, cars, and water. Canadians considered that insular thinking. There is much to question. Decisions on Mexico and Latin America also amounted to political football engineered by the president. The latest is the capture of the Latin American children from their mothers, never to see many of them again, causing worldwide wrath. The building of the wall between the two countries was another travesty. It would have been better to use that great deal of money to build a new sewage system between Tijuana, Mexico, and San Diego, California. It's a disgrace the way it is now and is far more than the Mexicans can afford to build alone. The sewage enters the Pacific Ocean and floats towards beautiful San Diego, causing disease and even death I've heard of many American sailors who did exercises in the contaminated water.

I'm afraid these are only a few problems Joe Biden and the new government will have to confront and work through. Some say the country is in chaos—that the numbers elected are too close and have been for some time. President Biden did such a good job getting a medical plan started in the US. Had the Republicans won the election, that may have been taken away. They think looking after health needs isn't democratic, even though almost every major nation in the world has plans for its citizens.

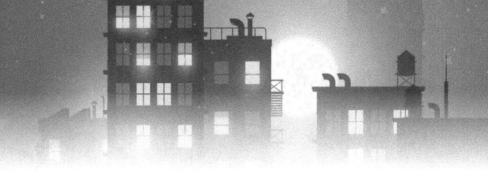

CABIN FEVER

Cabin fever from staying home so much because of COVID reminds me of a Charlie Chaplin movie called *Alaska*, I think. I loved Charlie Chaplin—even the ones made before talking motion pictures. He was so funny. You're probably too young for that movie; even I am, but I used to have copies of his movies until my daughter decided they had to go. I lost them in a cleanup of books, films, and records to the charity shop but if you're lucky, you might pick it up.

Although the crew of that silent movie *Alaska* is gone, the views and laughs linger on. In my mind, throughout these days of being confined, is the hope of getting COVID-19 numbers down in British Columbia. Compared to other jurisdictions, our numbers may be considered low, but we're in the second increase which must be dealt with this fall and winter until we have an injection that will protect us from the pandemic.

It was announced on the radio and TV that a shot that is said to be 90 percent protective to keep us safe is on its way so we won't get the virus again. Of course, with my luck, withdrawing the lucky number, I was never one to win even if it was a chance in five never in a million to one or 10 percent chance. However, we're all waiting for the day and will stay out of crowds, and I'll wear my face mask if that's what it takes.

I've watched enough TV this year that I'm sure the ratings must have gone up; even my remarks went on Knowledge Network. I've travelled around the world with Bill Murray's camera and Ken Burns films, of course, and many more travellers who have made it on Knowledge Network. I travelled around the world in my younger years—down the very streets they are now filming. I crossed that ocean that they are sailing on, took pictures of those very palm trees waving on Hawaiian beaches, and gazed at Mount Fuji, which is still looking like an ice cream cone. I saw Mexico's perimeters, just as mysterious, and Iceland from above. I know that my niece and her husband are down there on a mission for eighteen months. I pray that they are safe from COVID. We don't hear much from there about its spread. I could go on, but this isn't a travelogue per se. We all regret the passing of Alex Trebeck on the program, *Jeopardy*. He died of pancreatic cancer, though, not COVID. He suffered for a long time.

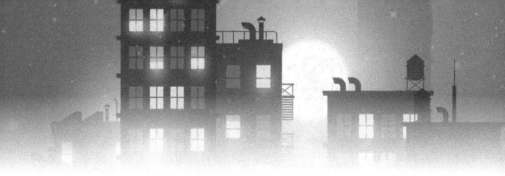

RESTRICTIONS

The biggest restrictions are still that the border is closed between Canada & the US. Not being able to cross the border into the US is really crippling to Canadians. A large percent of us like to head south for the whole winter. In fact, if we stay more than seven months, we'll be charged federal income taxes. In spite of the fact that we enjoy our motor homes, our winter home or campground. Others fly to Mexico, Florida, Cuba—you name it. Anywhere warm. That's also out of the question, although my granddaughter and husband went down to the Bahamas at the beginning of the pandemic. When they came back, they couldn't go back to work but had to go into quarantine for fourteen days. I'm sure they missed those paycheques.

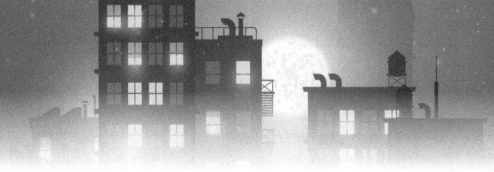

THE NEW NORMAL

Success means having the courage, the determination, and the will to become the person you believe you were meant to be.

—George Ryan

Stress and anxieties. Shortage of toilet paper and other things getting in short supply. It's silly, but it's real. "Climb every mountain. Ford every stream, follow every rainbow till you find your dream." I think everyone enjoyed that film.

Another singer, star actor, and member of the Latter-Day Saints Church, is Donny Osmond. I remember going to England one winter to see my husband's family and were they ever excited to get me in front of the telly and to see this little guy all dressed up in his little suit and up on stage with his brothers singing their hearts out. The family enjoyed them I could tell and the surprise was, as they pointed out was that they were over in Britain from their home in Salt Lake City and belonged to the same church I did. I've since seen them all on TV and on stage, including their one little sister, Marie. I don't think there is any other group that is watched and judged by the way they live as they are. It was much later that I saw Donny as the star in the Orpheum Theatre in Vancouver in Joseph's Coat of Many Colours, the story of Joseph in the Bible. I've got the name a little wrong. It is known as *Joseph's Multi-Colored Dream Coat.*

I express how much people look to other people as examples. Not everyone can be a great singer, piano player, or mathematician. Whatever you do, you should do your best. COVID may be trying at times, but when you get downhearted you might want to sing the song "You Raised Me Up." That's what Donny used to do

EVERYTHING IS POSSIBLE

Getting back to self-reliance, I will give you some suggestions that have worked for others, as they may work for you. If you have trouble doing this next step, you'll have to do something or stay the way you are.

This idea might help you. I hate the word *budget*, so call it what you will; it's to help you. It also depends on how you get paid, regularly every week, every month, time of sale, when the job is done, or whatever. Let's go! List all your proposed expenses for the year, including your once-a-year expenses. Don't know? Guess. You will have to do the math, as you may be short.

The Canadian government figured people spent all their paycheques every week, so they gave everyone one week's pay. Millions of people were losing their jobs, losing their businesses, changing their lives. Millions of people had lost members of their families and were forced to make decisions—big decisions. I have said the first thing to do is "pay your credit card down to zero and keep it there unless you like to pay as high as 29 percent interest. It grows like dandelions and when it gets you in its grasp, it's like having a noose around your neck—impossible to get free. There is no Lone Ranger to come along on horseback and save you.

Secondly, it's important to save enough money for a rainy day, as I've said before. Unless you like pandemics or think it's going to end tomorrow. More importantly, hang on to what you have. Spend only what you absolutely have to. You may be like the people in the news and face a forest fire or an earthquake or a war, heaven forbid. Be thankful if, by chance, your life is normal.

Get a good accounting system and change your life. You might wish to take courses, or return to college or night school, get help from family or knowledgeable acquaintances or professionals, whatever it takes. With the digital devices of today, you are far ahead of us old-timers. Some of us don't know a debit from a credit.

There is no magic in this pandemic. Some people are seeing things as they want to see it. You may have more money than your father gave you . . . I can say that as I never knew who my father was until this year. He would be approximately one hundred and twenty-five years old if he were alive today. Just as Matt Damon said about acting, "Work with the best director you can find." Find your director and do your best.

The magic (let's say "reality) is found and becomes real when you are lying in a bed in a hospital with tubes up your nose, a nurse at the side of the bed, a doctor somewhere in the building, your dad crying at home, hoping he won't get COVID, even sending up prayers that are emphatic, full of woe for your situation. Regretting every sin they ever conceived, wanting to see their father, praying that they haven't got COVID. "Let it be something else. God, have you forsaken me? Will Mother get it too and leave us? Will I be able to get back to school? Can I play outside? Should I keep it a secret? Is it too late to get an inoculation? Does Grandma know? Why doesn't she come to see me? I am anxious. I have no peace."

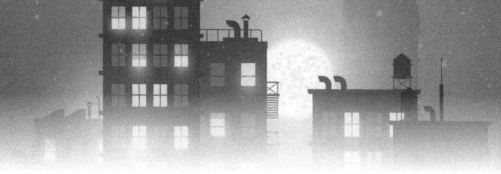

RETURN OF THE ANTS

My amazement at ants never left. How would a grown woman be charmed by them? It must have been the utter satisfaction with the ants in my bathroom of having actual living things in this time of utter isolation. Some people have a cat or a dog, and you can see them on television doing such smart tricks now that the owners have time to teach them with patience and rewards. Ants don't seem up for tricks, but they are still smart. One day when I entered the bathroom, I was amazed to find my friends the ants had piled tiny bits of fluff and dust in the corner by the bathtub. It was as if they had other fish to fry, as they had gone. It was late that I found a few of the tiny creatures on my cookstove. *Oh no!* I thought.

KNOWLEDGE BY ACCIDENT

This article came from CBC. It is definitely not complete but important, I think you will agree. It was on the radio this morning. You know I'm not too enthusiastic about CBC.

BE KIND, BE CALM, BE SAFE

Those were expressions given by Doctor Bonnie Henry in her book by the same name. I had never heard those three words strung together before. Had we been involved in all those broadcasts she gave and accepted the rules suggested by her and other doctors around the world during COVID, it perhaps (read: definitely) would be easier to prepare for and destroy this pandemic better, quicker, resulting in fewer people with the disease and far fewer casualties. I pray that you all are kind to your fellow human beings, being calm and not getting angry if things don't go your way, and obey the rules set down for you and everyone else. Many of the medical expressions she used in her book have become everyday English.

I thought flu shots covered everything. I was involved with any kind of medical threats that came my way. I guess I've been healthy most of my life. I got my shots and had I got SARS or any other strain going by I would have been like many others and would blame it on the shots from time to time, including pneumonia and shots when

I was about to go abroad, but I never thought that you could catch anything else; I thought it covered everything. I knew lots of people never got any shots. Boy, would they get a surprise if they came down with something floating around. I do remember while my husband was in the Royal Canadian Navy, he was taking a refresher course at Cornwallis, Nova Scotia, and fellow sailors were getting the flu but it wasn't the usual kind. They were sicker than a dog with rabies, as the saying goes. They couldn't eat. They just lay in their bunks and suffered in agony. Many died. That would have been about 1953, so many of you wouldn't remember it, and it's hoped that it will never come again. The doctors of today would be horrified that the guys on the course were subjected to those with such a contagious disease, knowing that it could have gone back to those on course and then back to an unbelievable number of families. By some miracle, although we were in Halifax, the children, my husband, and I didn't get it. I'll bet though that it was written up in the annals of Canadian history.

When SARS was around, I don't remember any restrictions like there are today. You just got it or you didn't. I imagine I would be shocked if I looked it up. I wonder what Google has to say about it. Maybe we're not doing enough to halt the spread of COVID-19. Maybe that's why many people say they aren't going to have an inoculation when it's invented and when it's offered. They're beginning to report that the inoculations may be invented in less time than expected. I'm sure they expect everyone to get their shots. I'll be at the front of the line if they let me.

In the meantime, it seems to be spreading all around the world. No country seems immune. Italy is one country that's being hardest hit. The United States seems not to take things seriously with the 2020 elections right around the corner although some experts are very aware but not too well taken seriously even though COVID has been with us for more than nine months. If inoculations are invented in less time than expected, they don't know yet who will get the shots first. Perhaps it will be the elderly, as they don't have the immune system to fight COVID . . . or maybe the health providers who are fighting it every day. And what countries will receive the vaccine first? I hope it's Canada, but maybe it will be the country that first comes up with the shots. Maybe it will be the countries that are suffering the most or the most congested like India or Great Britain. I understand the Prime Minister of Great Britain has already had the virus. The United States seems to ignore isolation norms.

Everywhere, hospitals are full. They don't have enough respirators; ordinary surgeries aren't being performed, and ultrasounds are on hold. When I had my knee replacement, I had a two-year wait. That was *before* the pandemic. The medical reception has been trying to catch up ever since. Also, nurses are unhappy about their working conditions, and specialists are scarce. Mine told me he was about to retire within seven years, and there are many more like him. I've had a conversation with my doctor once this year. It seems to be the new norm—a telephone call. I shall have to wait sometime to see her or get my x-rays.

THE MORE KNOWLEDGE YOU HAVE, THE BETTER YOU WILL BE ABLE TOFIGHT COVID NOW— AND SOLVE PROBLEMS IN THE FUTURE

Nelson Mandela—yes, the one from South Africa—once said, "I learned that courage wasn't the absence of fear but the triumph over it. The brave man is not he who does not feel afraid, but he who conquers that fear."

KNOWLEDGE BY ACCIDENT

Knowledge comes in all sorts of forms and may not be complete. The article that came across CBC radio this morning was certainly in that category. I'm not too enthusiastic about them since they didn't pay me or return my work, but I have appeared briefly on their TV program when I was promoting my first book, *Finding My Family*, but I should forgive them. The speaker spoke to us from a university in California. His name, if I heard it right, was Carlos Amedeo Ayanga. They spoke of a new name for an old feeling many of us are suffering from this pandemic we are going through which he referred to as *sosobra* in Spanish. Between himself and the CBC interpreter, the word *existentialism* was used.

It represented many of us who have uncertainty about the very ground we're standing on, a feeling of helplessness, a feeling of hopelessness, and anxiety. He also had the answer: if you don't want to suffer, the only freedom we have is *love*.

I knew a person in my own life who definitely fitted the portrait of this kind of personality. I hurriedly phoned him and bravely told him what I had heard and learned. I boldly spoke about the way he was living, not making decisions, feeling helpless, hopeless and watching his life pass him by.

When I said it was love that made the difference, he agreed with everything I had heard. I hope his life will be changed.

You, too, may be able to change someone else's life. I think of it myself when I get a bit depressed.

"Don't let COVID get you down. Follow the rules, love one another, and look forward and upward every day."

As for myself, I have no trouble making decisions in a hurry. However, I will carefully consider the future. For example, one time, my husband and I were looking at a house we wanted to buy. I wasn't sure what it was worth exactly, so I hesitated. The owner listed exactly the money she needed to have before she could sell. She listed the obligations she would have to pay when it was sold. When she was finished, I realized that it sounded reasonable, and for me, it would mean just a few extra mortgage payments down the road, so within minutes, I agreed. We bought it as is and where is and for the amount she wanted—no bargaining, no arguing. She was happy and I was happy. She was now free of her troubles, and I had bought a very unusual house with a monkey tree upfront. I was never sorry. I do know of those depressing thoughts first mentioned. Yes, I have made wrong decisions, but I worked through them over the years. And yes, I love people generally and that has a lot to do with it.

In these days of COVID, being confined to the house, not able to have anyone close due to the threat that wretched plague could infect me and all those I love dearly. They say that, at my age, I'm far more vulnerable. It's creepy, really. The number of patients entering hospitals and dying is going up every day no matter what we do. However, rumours have it that a vaccine will soon be ready in many countries. They just have to test it. It's a miracle actually, as many feared that it might take years. We should all be thankful. Of course, we're all in a line. Who will be the first to get it is another question and what will be the results be?

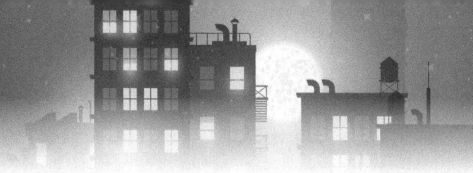

CHRISTMAS IN VIENNA
BROADCAST

N ever did I enjoy a broadcast as I did this one. But first a bit of my own to you in my poor Española:

FELIZ NAVIDAD *dos anno*
I want to wish you a Merry Christmas.
Espero anos
Silent night, holy night
Son of God, loves pure light
Jesus, Lord of our birth,
Sleep in heavenly peace.

I was inspired to write this piece about Christmas, as I noticed that some of the audience hadn't even clapped when the orchestra finished a most difficult piece. I surmised, maybe incorrectly, that they hadn't enjoyed it, and I couldn't help but wonder why. It probably wasn't a live concert, as people—even orchestra members—haven't been allowed to congregate in large numbers. Europeans are great supporters of musical events. I can picture them in their beautiful, immense opera houses during the winter and the thousands on the hillsides of the countryside in summertime enjoying the evening with their children. I surmised in this case that they didn't understand the music or were watching hours of music on television that didn't have a real audience where they wouldn't clap because they were the only ones set artificially. These days, it's difficult to tell. When we can go to a concert again after COVID, we may have to teach our children that they should clap at certain times and not at others.

I had never seen a real symphony concert until I was about ten years old, and I had no idea what was going on but was warned by my mother that I had to sit still and listen. I would guess that she had never seen a symphony before either; we had been invited by George and Alma Hammond, whom we lived with, to this concert put on by the Winnipeg Symphony Orchestra on the exhibition grounds of the Armoury building. I would say that few spectators had ever been to such a concert, and as the evening wore on, people got up and left the building. Mother whispered how that was very naughty, and we all stayed to the end. She had a saying, "If you can't clap because you enjoyed it, clap because it's over." I have heeded that advice ever since, and fortunately, my knowledge of fine music has increased over the years, starting in high school with our music teacher, whose name I have forgotten. I do remember that the kids said that the boys playing the trumpets were the best kissers. You never know what will come out of students' mouths. Teens haven't changed much in that regard.

COVID has limited most live concerts. Most are taped from days gone by. We are thankful that they are still here. The more education people have, the better the world will be. Fortunately, the schools are open. Children are wearing masks, and the classes are smaller, but in Canada, at least, it has been found that the younger people aren't so affected by COVID and when they do catch it, they don't seem to have the terrible results of the older folk.

Christmas will be lonely this year. For our own safety, we're encouraged not to even have relatives to Christmas dinner—nor can we have any parties, weddings, or funerals . . . not even church services. I can get Sunday morning church on the telephone or on *Zoom*. My friend Maryanne helps me get connected when I call. My technical skills are minimal at best. Recently I had over 900 messages waiting to be read on email. I got many read in a day—some from relatives, some from friends, but mostly advertisements of one kind or another. My son Douglas eliminated most of them, but they started coming back after twenty days or so. I get rid of some myself, but they come back before I draw breath.

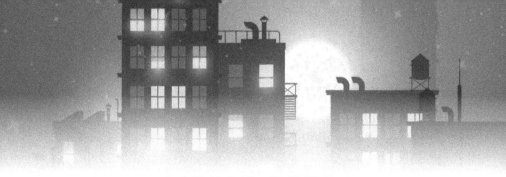

LITTLE PETS

Things get pretty tiring stuck at home day after day—no friends, no family, no hugs, no kisses. When will COVID be over? I'm no exception. I try to keep busy every day, making my bed and washing the dishes. Doing ordinary things, including writing books. It seems to sharpen my brain. The more I type, the more it seems to improve. What if that was the cure for Alzheimer's disease? Wouldn't that be wonderful? However, you couldn't just sit at home thinking about it. I've thought often of having a cat or a puppy perhaps. In the meantime, I have little beasties in the house recently. One little furry beasty I call Fuzzie. I would prefer a cat over a puppy because the cat may be able to cut down on all the fuzzies who seem to be able to scurry into the house even under a space as small as a pencil. They scurry across the floor and disappear behind the stove in the kitchen. I had stopped my rodent control service, as it was so expensive, and I've been trying to save for a new roof. However, common sense prevailed, and I called Robert at the pest control company. He came and explained why he was necessary to keep the little nasties under control, costly or not. He even found two mice in one trap on three occasions. One of these traps was behind my antique Chinese screen. At least they have good taste, but the female sex is generally terrified of mice, and I'm no exception. A strong male is needed in every house, but I understand that over age seventy, there are fifteen women to every man, so I'll have to wait for a superhero. I don't think my odds are too good. I should settle for a cat anyway to cuddle and talk to. However, they don't like to be left alone—except to sleep—and when COVID is beaten, I hope I can travel to all the places I'm now missing. In the meantime, I will settle for family's phone calls remembering that "Long conversations keep you from getting your work done."

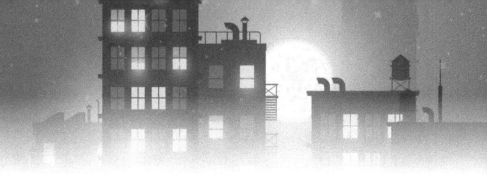

GRANDMA CURD'S CHRISTMAS 2020

DEDICATED TO GRANDCHILDREN EVERYWHERE

Well, as you might know, I'm confined to my home this Christmas for my protection from the pandemic, which will be worse if we have our family and loved ones spreading the disease around. However, we can keep in touch by telephone, cell phone or Internet, all of which are wonderful and getting better all the time. This Granma loves to visit with my grandchildren, and I'm grateful to have so many grandchildren and because we can't be together this year, I have chosen to write you this story of what happened:

I love writing stories. Don't you? This will not be a "once upon a time" story, though I love them, too—especially when it says at the end "And they lived happily ever after." I'll try to give this story a surprise ending. Let's see.

My story started about two weeks ago when I was dropping by to see my friend Zora in her backyard. We chose to meet there because of COVID so we would have fresh air and could stay two metres apart. I seldom visit, but being isolated, we like to keep in touch on the phone.

As we talked in the backyard and petted her dog, Winnie, we gazed up the street where some little men were reroofing a neighbour's house. *Click, click* went their hammers, and so cleverly, they went up and down the ladder while one helper helped by holding the big ladder from the ground. The house was beginning to look like new and ready for the holidays for the Christmas lights. It reminded me that my house needed roof work as well.

Winter was on its way, and the shingles on the roof would surely blow off if a bad storm came along, as those shingles had been on my roof for a long, long time. The roof had already lost many shingles in the past—many winters of small repairs. It shouldn't be neglected any longer.

Zora said she would see who the workers were and see if they could make mine look brand new like her neighbour's.

Sure enough, a few days later, I got a phone call from Top of the World Roofing Company. They could do my roof for me before Christmas if the weather stayed as good as it had been the last few days. No rain, but it was already December at this time of year, so it could also snow. That would mean they couldn't work. In Alberta, they already had lots and lots of snow.

The man who came to the house explained how badly neglected our house had been and what needed to be done. The work was extensive, but his helpers were good workers and would make it better than new. He remarked about how the house had been patched and patched but it was an old house and had a very sad roof. It could have loose shingles, which could blow away when the wind blew and the rain could get into the house, causing great damage.

He said he could start next week if the good weather held and he would guarantee his work.

Grandma was delighted! She said, "Go ahead!"

Sure enough, the following Monday, a huge truck arrived, and the helpers got busy unloading brand-new materials for the roof. The truck then headed to their next stop like Santa on Christmas Eve, but the man in the truck didn't have toys of course.

The very next day after the truck arrived, three helpers arrived and they set up the ladders and got busy unloading brand new materials for the roof. The truck headed to his next stop to help some other people. The helpers were bundled up like men from the North Pole with fluffy jackets, and fluffy pants to keep out the cold weather and the rain, even snow if it came down, hats that covered their ears with fluffy jackets and padded pants to keep out the cold, COVID masks for protection, gloves to keep their hands warm and cozy. They all seemed happy as they bustled up the ladders and started their job of renewing Grandma's roof.

TAP, TAP, TAP, all day long, those busy little men hammered loud and strong. The day had looked like rain. The sky looked grumbly with grey streaks and clouds in the distance. However, despite being grey, it didn't rain, and by 4 o'clock, a small section was done. The back and front porch looked better already.

> *TAP, TAP, TAP*, loud and strong,
> Time to go now seemed their song.
> Rain was forecast the next day,
> Maybe a big tent we'd need to borrow,
> But no, I'm happy to tell,
> Things went well all day long.
> *TAP, TAP, TAP*, it takes a long time,
> To fix our poor roof in British Columbia.

The wee men were getting like Santa's helpers more every day,
So busy and hard-working without delay.
Saturday it rained, but that was okay.
THE LITTLE MEN HAD A HOLIDAY
Sunday, too, for church and rest.
Every day they did their best.
Second week, boy this is quite a job,
Time to roast marshmallows on the hob.
The hob is the fire, but I was just fooling.
Monday came and the children they're schooling.
No time for watching the wee little men.
TAP, TAP, TAP, on and on they went
Grandma was sure they were Heaven-sent.
Christmas was just five days away
If it isn't finished what will Santa say?
Don't worry, said Grandma, scratching her head.
Maybe Santa can come down through a hole instead.
"No Grandma, but what if it rains?" a little voice said
"That will be a terrible dread."
"The ginger cookies would be mush instead."
"I was just kidding, now hop into bed."
"It will be done next week instead."
"And our little roofers can take a rest."
"And help Father Christmas do his best"
"To visit all the children who have gone to bed."
And Grandma will say, "This is the best "Christmas ever
Even if she says that every year forever.

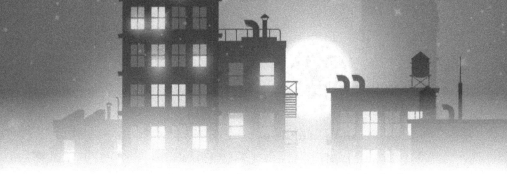

JEWISH HOLIDAY 2020

Many people in our city and certainly in Canada are Jewish and today on the Canadian Broadcasting Circuit I thought I heard that this year, both holidays coincide. I was quite impressed with the rituals they have to go through to make this time of year enjoyable. The only thing I remember as a child was that they put candles in the window. Actually, that put the family in danger because everyone would know they were Jewish. Thinking back, I would have said they were very brave with Hitler and his sympathizers breathing down their necks. Hatred is a terrible thing. Why do I mention it in a COVID year like this one? Well, it came back to me when there are so many people who will not get a COVID shot. They would rather die of the pandemic than do so, even if they take millions along with them. They may not hate any fraction of our population, but they surely hate anyone who thinks differently than them.

I mull about things like that now that I am confined to the house. I think of the troubles people of mixed blood have—and people of mixed marriages. I'm sure Jews don't discourage Christians from worshipping the birth of the Savior because He was the greatest of the Jews and, as Christians, we read the Old Testament as we do the New Testament. I reflect upon their holidays too that are based upon when the families put a mark on the door and those who were about to destroy the Jewish children passed them by and didn't destroy them. That Herod was a terrible man.

I also remember when Moses was leading them across the desert and God provided manna for them to eat. I always liked to hear about how Jonah was swallowed by the whale and the whale regurgitated him and many more events, good and bad, in the King James Version of the Old Testament in Sunday school—including when Job's wife looked back and was killed and, most of all, how Moses received the ten commandments, which are still relevant to everyone today. There is much, much more, but I don't know about their holidays, and if I judged anyone, it would be said, "She, (meaning me) is wanting. Now, getting back to Christmas, I wish we could all celebrate it together every year.

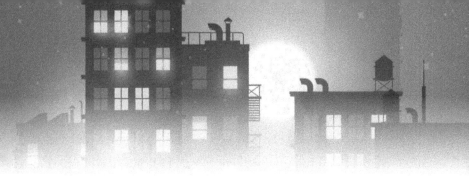

GRANDMA'S STORY OF
CHRISTMAS ON THE FARM

When our children were young and we lived on the farm I could talk about Charlie Brown's Christmas tree, but I think I have a real story you will enjoy:

We had just moved to a five-acre chicken farm in Cloverdale, and this was our first Christmas. Our oldest son, Maynard, was at Lord Tweedsmere High school in grade eight. It was a long way away, but he walked to school and back every day. Douglas was in grade five, and Glenna was in grade three. They were at Clayton School, and it was quite far too but not nearly as far away as their big brother's. They walked to school as well—there and back—every day. They all loved school. Glenna was one of the youngest in her class. They were so excited when Christmas was coming and they would have Christmas holidays. Letters were sent to Santa in the neighbourhood, and the Christmas concert was given at church with all the trimmings.

On the last day, the children came home with their report cards, and Douglas walked home with the class Christmas tree as they were all finished with it for another year. It was four days until Christmas. When I asked him how he got the tree, he said the teacher asked, "Who doesn't have a Christmas tree and would like one?" I shot up my hand, and she said I could have it if I could get it all the way home."

Oh, he was so proud of that tree. It didn't have any fancy globes left on it, but here and there were bits of silver icicles hanging here and there. It had its own wooden stand, so we put it up beside our black-and-white television in the living room not far from the oil heater, which too had a prominent place in the room and was our answer to the heating system for the whole house except for the oil range in the kitchen. For those who know about Charlie Brown's Christmas tree, this one closely resembled it.

A box of bobbles that were brought out of storage and a few ornaments of yesterday, as the saying goes, plus stars and snowflakes cut from coloured paper and brought home from school and a string of coloured lights that made the room shine (as long as not even one light went out) was draped on its branches. If one light went out, the whole tree went out, strange but true. Just ask Grandpa.

That was not all. There was an angel for up top, and it was wafted into place with more silver icicles put on by the children. "Oh, it's so beautiful!" we all agreed.

"Time for sleep, children. The night is here."

All were soon fast asleep. Oh, I forgot about our black and white cat that we called Sylvester. He shared our life and was pretty well the boss of the house. He was a wonderful pet—until that night, that is. Apparently, he loved the tree as much as we did. All of a sudden, a huge crash was heard. I was awake in a start.

"Oh no!" It took only a minute or two to realize what the cat had been up to. Obviously, he had seen the tree and thought to himself, *What a wonderful chance I have to climb into its beautiful branches.* And up he went. Crash went the tree. Down went our wonderful Charlie Brown Christmas tree. Crash went the bobbles, leaving little pieces of glass all over the floor. Crash went the needles on the tree as they were already dry, having been not only in our house but a week in the schoolroom as well and had become dry as toast, as Grandma would say. The cat had run away to hide in the kitchen corner behind the cook stove.

Our sleepy eyes decided that sleeping was better than cleaning up all that mess in the middle of the night, so I suggested that we all go back to bed and worry about the mess in the morning. Not one person objected to that idea, and we all went back to our rooms.

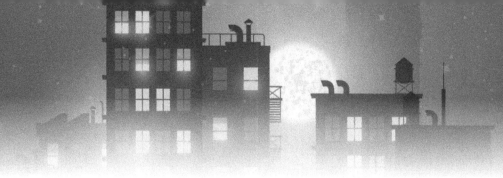

INFECTIONS 2020

I t was just announced today that because so many people in Canada had their flu shot, there were no reported deaths from flu-related illnesses. That was amazing. Of course, they added that we had obeyed the COVID regulations, staying at home if you felt ill, having your flu shots, and staying away from others. Now, if we obey those rules in 2021 and get the vaccine, we can expect to beat this noxious plague. That came across on the radio on December 28, 2020, according to my journal. However, it doesn't mention that a vaccine for everyone is very slow in coming. It also mentioned a Richard Strouse concert is coming from Vienna tonight. It can hardly be expected to be a live concert but one taped maybe several years ago. No audience will be in attendance. I know it will still be wonderful or as we say in Vienna . . . wonderbar.

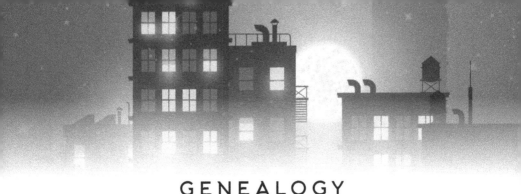

GENEALOGY

I t's not every day that people will tell you they have found their father and life goes on. COVID or no COVID, this morning, my son Douglas phoned to tell me that he had found my grandfather and he had a phone number to call in order to find out who my father probably was. I knew he had been working on the family genealogy for a long time, but I hadn't realized how serious it had become. He had asked me many questions about my sister Dorothy's family, and I had given him names of his cousins in that family and some of the telephone numbers but I didn't think that would help.

I had searched for many years and found scads of family trees, especially after I had found my brothers and sisters. However, genealogy has become easier with technology and especially with DNA—and more and more accurate tests are available. It's incredible! My sister and I had been brought up without any relatives, or so we thought. I wrote about it in my first book, *Finding My Family*. Our mother kept the past to herself. In fact, she went to her grave without revealing her past.

I had my suspicions and eventually found my siblings—ten living, in fact, through a simple conversation my husband had with her about the old days. She unknowingly let something fall from her lips that I was able to put into context and by putting the pieces together, we were able to find people from her past who led us to a brother-in-law in her past and so to her children (our brothers and sisters) less than a hundred miles from my home in Vancouver where they had been all the time. They, in turn, told of Mother having received money from a mutual friend of our parents which led to their separation. According to the children, Mother was so angry that she opened up the stove lid and threw the money in the fire. The children all remembered how big their eyes went when that happened at a time when money was so scarce in their family. When she left, she had made arrangements to take Aggie, the oldest, and Clarence, the youngest, but Aggie wouldn't go, and Mother couldn't work and look after Clarence. Aggie stayed with her brother and sisters. They were Ethel, Ruby, Helen, Wilfred, Dora, and Belle, adding up to eight children in all.

They talked about her coming back and visiting with those who caught Scarlet Fever and ended up in the hospital. That was somewhat like the COVID of the '20s. It was very contagious and serious. Fortunately, no one around them died.

When I found the family, they were so happy that after forty-one years, I was able to do so. Dora had come very close to finding us when I was in grade eight or thereabouts. I remember the day a policeman came to our door on McIntyre St. Mother wouldn't tell me what he wanted when I asked her. I was curious, but she would never say.

Many years have gone by, and most recently, my son Douglas got interested in genealogy. He also found that, with the pandemic, he had time on his hands when he couldn't travel or visit with his relatives. He traced the Hogg side of the family back to a king of England way back when—not quite to Adam and Eve. He worked with his cousins but was finding things didn't always work out. Sometimes, he would be related to one cousin and not another. More and more of the finding didn't make sense. It was fun to find and talk to all these new relatives, but finding out how they fit in was another problem. If they were on my mother's side, everything went together. He was getting replies from England, Finland—even Australia—but they didn't come back on the Ray (Wray) or Day line. Instead, it would come back on Mother's side. Doug was perplexed. He started questioning me on my side about who my grandmother's family was. No luck. In the meantime, he was helping a lady in Norfolk, England. This was getting exciting! He got us all connected up on the computer, and we were able to talk to each other. A beautiful young lady looked back at me. She looked an awful like I was looking in a mirror many years ago. She had blond hair, not snow white like mine is today. She had the same nose (nobody has a nose like mine). No wrinkles, of course, but blue eyes like mine. I guess from her point of view we didn't look a bit alike, and she didn't think there was any relationship, but what she had to say just about knocked my socks off. She said she had found my grandfather. She said his wife was Brown, and your father is one of two brothers, Alfred Charles Farrow or . . . I immediately stopped her. Oh, my goodness, I had known him all my life, but my mother hadn't told me, and he had never lived with us. I was all shaken up when I hung up the phone. She had told me the other brother's name, but I knew that Charlie was the one.

Yes, Charlie as we called him, not Alfred Charles as his real name was, but it was amazingly Charles on my birth certificate, although Mother had changed it to Charles Maynard. Don't ask me why; I do not know. Be that as it may, she remained married to Chester William Ray all her life, and he never remarried, but that was the argument back on the prairies that my brothers and sisters witnessed when Mother brought home the money and they had the fight over. Chester suspected her of cheating on him, and I guess if any of them were alive today, they could say "I told you so," and of course, science can newly prove it.

My brothers and sisters that I found when I was in my forties had told me that story, and the sister I grew up with, who was 2 and a half years younger than I, talks about the time the landlady gave us notice. I remember Charlie visiting us there and his big black woolly coat. I believe he continued to give us money to get through the Great Depression of the thirties. As an undertaker, he always drove a big black car which must have cost a lot of money and maybe it was large enough to transport the bodies of people who had died. Later on, when I was older, someone told me that times were so tough that he sometimes donated one of his suits for the funeral of a citizen. In his early days in Canada, he lived and ran a second-hand store in Sintaluta, Saskatchewan, but later, he purchased a beautiful home in Indian Head, where my girlfriend Eileen and I would go out to visit on weekends just to get away from the city. Eileen had a train pass because her father worked for the CP Railroad, so it was probably her idea in the first place. I never dreamed that he was anyone more than Uncle Charlie.

I remember he used to come to see us, and Mother would say, "Clear off a chair so Uncle Charley can sit down."

He never stayed long. Once he gave me a ride to Central Collegiate where I went to school. I could never forget it. I was so embarrassed at arriving in a hearse that I jumped out almost before it stopped in case some of the kids might see and make fun of me.

However, looking back, I think of times Mother sent us out to Lumsden on the train to spend holidays with Bertha Hamilton and her husband, Claude. If anyone asked, it was because she couldn't work and look after us at the same time.

My mind goes wild, and my imagination puts facts in my life, especially since my book "Finding My Family" has become known around the country. For example, when I contact people with the name Maynard, I think, *Could they be our brother?* We always wanted a brother. In my wildest imagination, I would think that Mother could have been pregnant during those holidays and being chubby all the time, we wouldn't have known. The dates involved working out, as Dorothy had been born after me. I received a letter from Alberta from a man who had read my book, and he said that he or someone in the family had the name Maynard, and they never knew where they got it. I still can't wait to see what my son Douglas finds by searching through DNA files. Another letter came from Southern Saskatchewan, though I have never mentioned my concerns to him, as I'm sure he will think it's ridiculous.

Dorothy and I were so happy when we found our brothers and sisters—and to find two brothers, Clarence and Wilfred.

We haven't even proven that Dorothy is my biological sister. She was so different than me in many ways. She had brown naturally curly hair. Mine was perfectly straight. Both of us had blue eyes—that I will admit. Dot was big-boned and much taller than me. Her bones were much stronger than mine. Her temperament was quite different and she got her way with Mom much more than I did. Her hands were much bigger than mine, and I'm sure, had we had the opportunity, she would have been much better on the piano. I was more studious, but she was the youngest in her class, so I'm sure that held her back. I'll admit that Charlie Farrow gave me more attention than he did Dot. He used to give me kisses when he came for a visit. I didn't like to be kissed. No one in my life ever kissed me, including my mother. He may have kissed my sister, but I cannot recall.

Charlie talked to me about his travels as I got older—how he went to funeral conventions in the US. He gave us an atlas, and I tried to memorize every state in the union and their capitals. I never dreamed at the time that I would visit almost every one of them—well, at least half—in my lifetime. He never mentioned higher education for me. I wish he had. Perhaps he thought I would be successful on my own, and I think you can say that I was. It took me a long time with the help of many people, but I'm thankful for all the education I had. I say this on a day when I'm more or less confined to home by COVID, and I share it all with you.

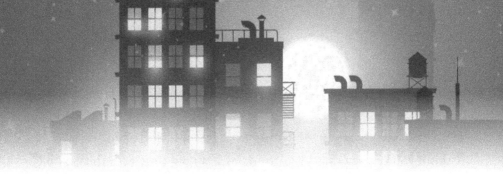

VACCINATIONS STARTED

JANUARY 4, 2021

It's been a rough road, but vaccinations for COVID have begun sooner than expected. Canada is ahead of the US—for now, anyway. Our doctors and caregivers are among the first to get their shots, along with indigenous groups and the elderly in care homes and others with the most need. The US is apparently having distribution problems. Serious problems. President Donald Trump doesn't seem to agree with certain actions that have been taken. They seem to persist. The news is so negative, and I thought I understood US politics. After all, I have US citizenship because my mother was American. I don't expect anyone to agree with me no matter how right I am (do I hear laughter?), but they need to knuckle down as their cases of COVID are climbing and climbing and people are dying.

I'm Canadian by birth, but most of my brothers and sisters are American by naturalization, as they were all born in Saskatchewan, Canada. They, too, are British subjects, as they were born before 1967, some in Riverhurst and some in Regina, all in Saskatchewan, Canada. I'm also a British subject by birth, a member of the British Empire. However, I like to think of myself as a citizen of the world because of all my travels. I spell like a Canadian (I guess you noticed that already, when I use the word *neighbour*, for instance).

I can even say I bumped into Donald Trump in Los Vegas once long before someone talked him into running for president. My husband, Charlie, had rushed over to me in the Bellagio and said, "Come with me and see who I have seen." It turned out to be Donald talking like he always does, sitting at a table in the next room not far from where the pianist keeps us all entertained with soft music while we feed the machines in that beautiful gambling den. "There's Donald Trump." Well, there he was at a table around the corner of the lobby, probably negotiating some deal there in Vegas. I bet he was smart enough not to gamble. I always wondered what he was cooking up. Maybe it was a new high-rise in Waikiki, Hawaii, as several years later, he built a high-rise not far from the ocean and took away my view of the beautiful Pacific from my hotel. I never forgave him for that. (Just kidding. If things were reversed, I might have done the same.)

When I heard Donald was running for president of the United States, I pictured him back at that table in Vegas brewing up some scheme, but this time they were talking about the upcoming election, which may have gone something like him being Republican saying a few snide remarks about President Obama and one of his cohorts saying, "Donald you should run for president." and another chirping in, "Yeh, why don't you run for president? You would win for sure. That would fix those Democrats."

Donald, being Donald, agreed it was a good idea. I can't imagine him giving it much thought. I wonder what his family said when they heard. Maybe someday we will know. I know I just shook my head when I heard, and I don't even have a vote. Strangely enough, I knew a lot of Americans liked him so I agreed that "Yes, he could win and down would go the medical system Obama tried so hard to set up."

We would go down south to California during the worst part of the winter in Canada in the motorhome. The fellow tourists would speak quite openly with me. Their prejudices against the Mexicans, the Blacks, and even the Canadians were quite pronounced once in a while. Not all Americans were like that, but it rather upset me. I always felt. "Cher la difference" is what I would say ("love the difference"). Latinos were no exception, and while travelling in Latin America, I tried to speak Spanish. I was never good at it. The thought of building a fence between the two borders didn't make sense. Tijuana, Mexico, desperately needs a sewage treatment plant. Now if the US Government had spent their dollars on that instead of a fence between the two countries, instead of a barrier, that may have made sense. They seemed oblivious to the fact that the sewage wasn't only destroying the lives of the Mexicans, but it was destroying those who worked for San Diego Sanitation and sailors in the US Navy, who were based in San Diego were being destroyed due to the pollution along that portion of the coast—especially those in training, not to mention the harm done to the beautiful San Diego Zoo and the visitors living between there and the border. I guess I'm growing old, and no country is perfect.

The Free Trade Agreement is another thorn in Donald Trump's side. He couldn't get rid of it fast enough. He didn't understand it, but he wanted it gone. I'd had a conversation with some Idahoans, who must have been Republicans, who wanted things changed because they wanted the cost of pork to be cheaper in Canada or some such nonsense. Well, they have it now. I hope they're happy. Other citizens in that state are sad about COVID because Canadians can no longer cross the border to shop.

My brother was a dairy farmer in Washington State, and we used to have these conversations together. He always thought that the gallons of milk should be cheaper in Canada because he never felt he was getting enough for his produce in the US. However, I noticed that he had the latest Cadillac, and the truck with the special compartment in the back that a Canadian farmer would be very envious of. I loved my brother Clarence and didn't begrudge anything he owned. He worked hard and took very few holidays. This has little to do with COVID, but it was his daughter, Crystal, who first told me about this strange "flu" that had put so many Washingtonians in the hospital before anyone in Canada ever heard of it.

Many Republicans were against Obamacare. They would make remarks like "But your medical is free in Canada." I don't know where they got that idea. Nothing in Canada is free. We pay through taxes just like we pay for our highways. One of my brothers-in-law in the states lost his house and practically everything he owned before he got help with his medical bills. I remember that having a baby in the States, especially a cesarean section, was so expensive for a young couple. I knew what that was like because I had three babies that way before we had a medical plan. We have Tommy Douglas to thank for our medical plan among thousands of others. It wasn't easy. One of my nieces in Washington State told me she is waiting until she's sixty-five before she has a much-needed operation. When I asked her why, she said that then she would be on Medicare. Pity.

Donald Trump wanted all the Mexican illegals to be kicked out of the country. He went as far as capturing those fleeing across from Central American countries because of the horrible conditions down there and separating them from their children. It was tragic, and many of those children weren't returned to their parents I heard.

Many people are wondering why the voting was so close in this 2020 election. A two-party system like that would never work in Canada. We presently have four parties—the Democrats, the Republicans, the NDP and The Green Party. I'm not saying it's easy.

I met an American lady complaining about the cars in the US, although this story could be told in Canada as well.

"They should make all the foreign companies go home."

"Why?" I asked.

"So there would be more jobs for Americans" she replied.

"Oh?" I said, "What kind of a car do you drive?"

"Japanese Toyota, of course," she replied.

"Oh, if you want them to stay across the ocean why did you buy a Japanese car?"

"Oh, it was cheaper and got more miles to the gallon."

End of story. I think you got the message. We have to stand behind what we believe in or not complain.

Now you can buy a hybrid or electric car, but the same rules apply.

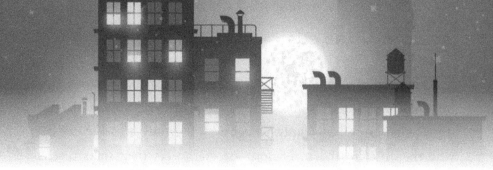

BACK TO COVID

JANUARY 15, 2021

Not much is happening being stuck at home. Staying away from the stores, avoiding people, no visitors, the odd business call, wearing masks, calls on the phone to everyone else (including family), a cell phone that doesn't work for me, church services online, my back sunroom with the washing machine in the background and a messy make-do office and the clothes dryer hoping for spring when we can hang the clothes out on the clothes rack to dry in the sunshine on the back porch.

It's more exciting in Washington, DC. However, I don't like that kind of excitement—even if it is Donald Trump about to be impeached because of the overtaking of the Capitol Building with him cheering them on in spite of the loss of life by the rioters instigated by Trump. It was no ordinary show of distaste but a real mob with guns, and other weapons, including furniture that had been destroyed and used as weapons, destruction of records and other papers, breakage of doors, and grabbing anything that could be used as a weapon. Then there was the breaking of windows while elected officials took cover as best they could. It was all on TV, and much more failed to be covered, including a woman and a police officer who were killed.

In spite of all the bad news, COVID vaccinations have arrived in Canada. Caregivers and indigenous people are among the first to get the serum. Obviously, caregivers are greatly at risk every day, and the different Indian Nations are due to get their shots first, as they considered the tightness of their living quarters. Those far from hospitals and ambulances or transportation are also at risk.

Next in line are the elderly, those over seventy like myself and those in senior homes where records have been dire, partly because in senior homes where records have been kept, there have been many deaths because many seniors live two or more to a room, and aides often go from one establishment to another, so the disease is easily spread.

Going back in history, I remember my mother didn't want to be put in a shared room when she got old but she didn't mind living in a small room—an extra-long hall closet, in fact, in a rooming house as long as she had it all to herself. She died before she had to face COVID. In many ways I am thankful. She was eighty-four.

Getting back to COVID and the inoculations, most of the population will have to wait until more serum has arrived and can be distributed. Until then, we're urged to stay apart from others as much as we can so we won't be stricken. It has made me uneasy to even leave the house. I want to go shopping, and I'll go out with the lady downstairs to buy groceries. I'm hesitating to go to the pharmacy (that is only imperative every three months for my tablets), but oh it would be nice to roam the aisles of the dollar store. I tell everyone that I don't drink and I don't smoke, so I can spend as much money as I like (once in a while) in the dollar store of my choice. Some agree. I also enjoy thrift stores or, as some may call them, "second-hand stores." You take stuff there and you buy some more. Right? The place I long for most perhaps is a local restaurant called White Spot. They make the best fish and chips with Zucchini on the side. (Yummy.) I can hardly wait. Now they may have become a takeout place.

The streets were deserted there for a while compared to normal, but the number of cars has seemed to pick up. Spring is here. Schools have reopened. Teachers are back. Parents in our neighbourhood seem to be driving the youngest to elementary on our corner. The kids are taught to keep their distance on the playground. It must be difficult. I'm not sure about masks, but they may even have to wear them in school as well. Young children aren't scheduled for vaccination. They don't seem to get COVID. My teaching days are over.

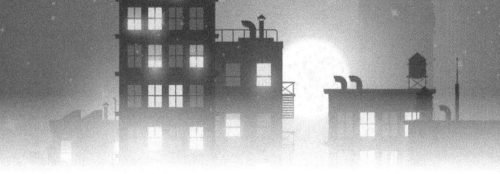

FINANCIALLY YOURS

Everyone has their own money problems during this pandemic, some good, some not so good, from getting rich to worse off than before. The government stepped in and helped many people and was criticized for doing so. I received $300.00 (approximately), and I was happy until someone explained to me why I got it. Landlords weren't able to raise the rents, which was a real good idea, but you know what side of the fence I'm on. Still, it was a good idea. Landlords had a bad habit of giving tenants two months' notice even if they had been there for twenty years and they would go in and refurbish the apartment or house and up the rents. In Vancouver, there is always a shortage of housing, so this wasn't a great idea during a pandemic.

Owners were forgiven their mortgage payments if they lost their jobs because of the pandemic, and interest rates were lowered at the banks. I'm trying to pay my line of credit down as fast as I can, as the bank has already told me it'll go back up after this is over. It means I must cut back as much as possible on everything. It's easy to cut back on travel, as we aren't allowed to travel out of the province—never mind the country. Common sense tells us that maybe that's a safe rule.

The homeless are perhaps the worst off in the country. There have been a few weak endeavours to help, but the number keeps growing. Also of note are the immigrants and refugees from other countries.

Canada has less than a 2 percent birthrate, so we can let many more people into the country, but they seem to be swamped with the paperwork. They don't know how to say "Come on in. We need you." I should complain, as my son worked keeping people out when he worked for the government. Obviously, it hasn't changed. Have you heard this expression? "Orders are orders!"

Some people are able to work at home, which is good. It keeps their car in the garage and them free from catching COVID from fellow workers. Other businesses have had to lay people off, and some have had to go out of business, which is a pity. No one knows when this is all going to end. Therefore, they live in fear and trepidation. Some companies are holding on in a wait-and-see situation.

As I'm amongst the retired population, nothing much has changed as far as what money I receive. However, expenses always seem to go up. They say groceries go up, but I haven't spent any more than before. You can manage as I'm determined to. I need shoes, mainly because I have to use gadgets to put my shoes on that definitely don't work on shoes that have ties or that fall off easily. I have to take two very expensive pills a day, and to save money, I sometimes took only one in the morning and none at night. This is definitely not recommended. I also ordered a three-month supply to avoid paying filling charges. I learned by experience that if I ran out early, the pharmacist charged to fill a three-day supply. That hurt. Also, I would have to pay three-month charges for each month unless I filled them as a group. The latest thing I learned was to shop around to get the best price. So far, I haven't resorted to that, as it's a difficult process with so few places that will deliver. It's not wise to not take all the pills prescribed. The moral of the story is this: "Be smart. I want you to learn from every experience."

1. Cell phones – Everyone in my life has a cell phone. I would not ask them to give them up. I have, but I haven't given mine up. I loved it, but I couldn't get my cell to open. Maybe later. (Complaints of an old lady.) People around me used to have to open it wherever I brought it.

2. I limited the use of the car – This was easy, as we were encouraged to stay home.

3. Bought bigger sizes at the grocery store – I shopped at an economy grocery store. However, specials can pop up anywhere. I stayed out of the mall to stay away from people, but it's such a tempting place. Let's just say I put it on the back burner.

4. Gave a cheque to charity instead of gifts to my son as a Christmas gift – A few years ago, he had done the same for me. My gift was a goat. Yes, I knew he wouldn't mind, and we made the people in Africa very happy. I had recently bought my great-grandchildren a gift I knew they would like. It cost $4.00 at the dollar store, but it turned out to cost $16.00 to mail it. Maybe next time it would be cheaper to send a cheque and let them spend it as they wish. I'm not quite sure about that.

5. I don't encourage anyone to buy online. On rare occasions, I have. I can see it can be addictive. The dress looked so beautiful, but an oversize is not like an eighteen, and I had to give it away to a friend who is much smaller than I.

I love it when things get mailed right to the door. Another problem was when I ordered four bottles of pills. They came, and when I opened them, the bottom of each bottle had pills in it, but I could have put them all into one bottle and saved the money. I wrote back to them but got no answer. The only thing left is to mail them back and pray they get them. All I can say is . . . BEWARE.

6. I wash all the clothes in cold water with gentle soap and dry them outside. Some neighbours may not like clothes out on the lines but my next door neighbours don't seem to mind. I've seen clothes on the patios too. but that, too, could be a problem.

7. I do use the dishwasher, but I try to get a large load to start, but I don't overdo it.

8. My granddaughter introduced me to energy-efficient garbage bags, as the green stuff is biodegradable and gets turned into soil.

9. I try to conserve everything, including hot water.

10. Last year, I had the heating system replaced. It was expensive, but over the coming years, it will pay for itself—or so I'm told. The gas bill has been showing a savings of 3 percent. Of course, that isn't a lot, but I had to have a new water heater anyway. Actually, I could have had a more efficient water heater, but I didn't think of it at the time. Years ago,

we had double-glazed windows put in our ancient house. We were encouraged to do so at the time. They said they would pay for themselves in a few years. As it turned out the day we got them, I was amazed by how quiet the house was. The noise from the cars had disappeared.

11. The roof was another matter. It, too, needed replacing. It would cost twice what the house cost sixty years ago. However, a winter storm could do great damage. It looks lovely and I feel secure. It is guaranteed forever (I gather that means the life of the house.)

12. Add your own way to save money every day.

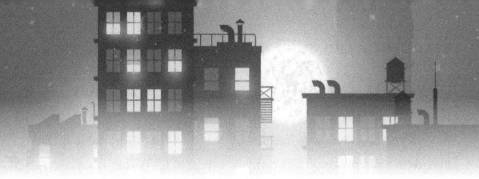

STORMING THE
CAPITOL BUILDING

They say Trump's action was anarchy in action in Washington, DC, in January 2020. What was he thinking? Did he feel that after all the checking of the ballot, they still hadn't been counted right and he was the rightful president of the United States? And what made him think he had the right to encourage vigilantes to tear down the Capitol Building and endanger so many people?

What is President Joe Biden inheriting when it's all over? Will Donald Trump be found guilty, and if he is, will he pay for all the damage done? It will be difficult with such a narrow margin of Democrats over Republicans to run the government. What were Donald Trump's followers thinking? What was their purpose? To destroy? To push? To kill anyone who got in their way, including members of the opposition? To destroy everything using sticks as weapons, or anything they could get their hands on as they climbed the walls on the outside and inside of the building? It certainly looked like it on television. All of this was being recorded on air if you can imagine. I know if my mother was still alive, she would be saying, "If someone tells you to jump in the river would you, do it? In other words, "If someone asks you to do something that isn't right, would you do it?" You will all go down in history for the wrong reasons and there may be others that follow you if you haven't learned.

What decisions will have to be made in the future with such a narrow-elected majority, especially at a time of COVID?

AUTOMOBILES DURING COVID

I had never owned a new car in my life. Fast forward and a year before COVID I found myself in a car sales operation. Some in the family thought my old car wasn't right for me. Looking back, I felt like I was a lamb being led to the slaughter. It was hated at first sight. I'm short, and I couldn't see over the wheel. The salesman adjusted it, but it was never right for me. It was made for someone much taller. It was so modern that I didn't understand the wipers or the temperature control, the left side, the right side, reverse, how the seats went down, the storage opening in the back—any of it.

The storage was small with little room for my walker without the back seat down, and the price was too high, though it wasn't discussed. Someone got a $500.00 cheque for bringing in the sale, but it wasn't me. The interest rate was a handsome zero percent, but when the last payment was made, almost the same month as COVID began, the price paid was certainly enormous. I thought that thirty-six months would never end.

Since COVID started, we're not encouraged to travel, so it was all sort of a payment for nothing plus insurance. We in British Columbia did so well, we did get a small refund, so that was a treat. We got it because there were fewer accidents during the year. Now if we could only do that every year.

January 17, 2021

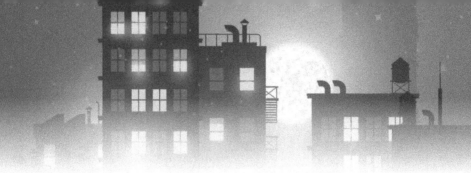

A NIGHTMARE TO REMEMBER

Many people report that they've been having nightmares lately. I've had dreams, but so far, nothing to be called a nightmare. My dreams usually leave as quickly as they come. I don't remember them in the morning. However, the dream I had last night was different.

In my dream, I was surrounded by work. The kitchen sink was piled up with dishes. I had the added things from baking a carrot cake (one way to get more veggies in my diet)—empty sugar jar, tins, tart pans, measuring cups, mixers, and tongs, cutlery . . . you name it. Breakfast dishes, snack dishes, garbage to go out. I planned to give the cake away, but I had forgotten the cream cheese for the icing. What's a carrot cake without the cream cheese icing? I wondered how I was going to eat two cakes alone? Well maybe with ice cream. I know it is not a good substitute, but after all, this is the pandemic. What a dream!

Next thing I knew, I saw my husband coming towards me. (I'm a widow but in the dream, I had a husband). He waved at me, surrounded by people. I felt helpless as I'd had a call from renters who were having trouble with their sheets of all things. (I don't even supply sheets.) I said that I would bring some over, but I was nearly in tears wondering how I could do all the work and look after them too. I tried to walk over on my own, but along the path, it was so muddy and difficult to navigate because of a rainstorm. Miraculously, my husband in the dream came and the path got easier. We arrived at the apartment. I can only remember that it was strange with high ceilings.

Sorry, but that's all I remember—my husband not helping me at first and then going with me. I can't even remember who the renters were, but they were there. I don't even know why it was important to tell you, the reader, but maybe because so many of us are alone. Perhaps I sympathize with those who have been having bad dreams these days and are afraid of what is happening around us—afraid we might break the rules, explaining the messed-up kitchen in the dream, and afraid we may not get our COVID shots before we mess up and not be protected. I've always felt as if my husband was my protection. Maybe food or the lack of food comes into it. There have been successes and setbacks with the shipment of supplies on occasion, and postponements. Some people say they don't even want the Covid shot, therefore endangering others, including me.

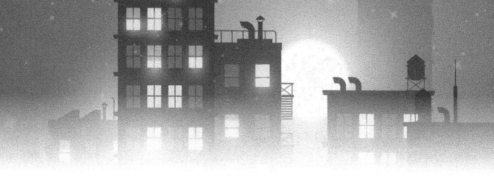

HOUSING

Here I am in my cozy house, but so many people are homeless—here in Vancouver, across Canada, and throughout the world. It's not just this year but has been getting worse year by year. The person, country, government or charity that can find the answer will go down in history. Every day I ask, "What can I do?" I have helped Habitat for Humanity but maybe not enough and have witnessed how municipalities have refused to give them building permits for years to keep them from building in their city. Herald all who have helped. I believe President Jimmy Carter was the one to get it started.

One of my friends helped build forty-five homes in Winnipeg a few years ago, but most of the futile answers have been provided by well-meaning governments who find it isn't in their interests to build for the less fortunate. They may not have answered at all or issued a response saying that permits were still "down the road." I can't say. It's better than nothing, although that's a terrible reply.

It can't be true, but I have heard that those on the street can't receive help from food banks, as they don't have a permanent address. Maybe someone will correct me.

In the meantime, vacancies in the city have doubled. I think I'm wrong about that as well. That would bring it up to 2 percent. For years, rentals have shown a 1 percent vacancy rate, which is a sad number, indeed. I think that it's a case of "The more money you have, the more opportunity you will have." Many need subsidized housing.

Vancouver is also one of the most expensive places to live in the world. In spite of the pandemic, housing isn't considered reasonable. Even those who have a roof over their head require to be fed, given health insurance, medicine perhaps, and clothing, and can we leave out a cellphone and Internet connection, along with electricity connection, heating, transportation, education, and the list goes on. I know that cellphones and the Internet are more expensive than in other places. I was offered a slight reduction on my phone if I would sign up for two years. I refused. My husband had signed up for two years and unfortunately died, and I was left to make the payments for two years.

Recently, in the last couple of years, it was broadcast that Internet and telephones would be reduced to $7.00. The companies may have received the new technology, but it may be a while before it floats down to the rest of us.

Present companies also seem to charge to discontinue your service to prevent mostly customers to move around to other companies.

February 2021

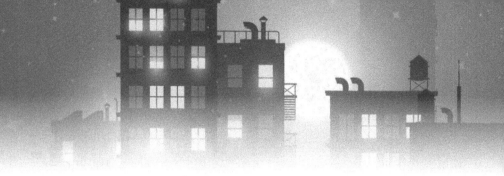

INOCULATIONS

When is it my turn? What does *freedom* mean? Well, as far as COVID is concerned, it means "When I get my COVID shot. That will mean freedom." (It has been approved, but now everyone in the country must fall in line to get one. When COVID-19 first started, it was predicted that it may take years, mainly based on how long it took before Dr. Salk came out with his wonderful vaccine to make polio a thing of the past. How many children were crippled for life before that happened? It is hard to tell. Will we ever be able to thank him and those who helped him? It took seventeen years before there was a success in the lab. How long would it take this time? The reckless predicted "months." The wiser weren't so sure and thought it could be years. Some people could be cured in one area and the pandemic could be rampaging somewhere else. It will take everyone to take the virus from spreading. My heart weeps when I think of it.

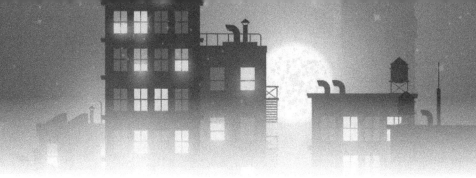

A NEW ERA

Actually, in Canada, the caregivers and some elderly care homes had received their COVID shots. However, there were many deaths before that. It's complicated, and there were as many reasons to celebrate the successes as there were to criticize the failure. That's often true in life. We hail the successes and blame the failures. That's where history comes in.

This is the day of ex-President Trump's impeachment trial. What seems clear is that he will be impeached for inciting the riot that led to the breaking of the windows and forcing their way into the Capitol Building in Washington, D.C. And the destruction and mayhem and deaths that they caused by his egging them on. It happened while he was still in office and is important because it is his second incitement and will prevent him from ever running again. In fact, I wonder what he would say if you asked him why he ran in the first place.

People tease me and say "Be careful what you tell Belle or it will end up in one of her books."

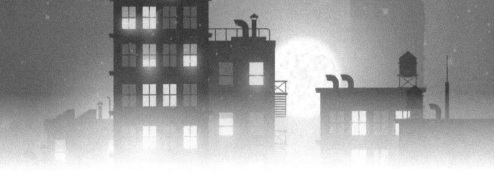

OUR GALAXY

We may think that we are alone in our galaxy or you are alone during quarantine. This past year, from January 2020 to January 2021, many people thought that we were alone in our galaxy as well. In 1895, the year my mother was born, who thought man could walk on the moon, that there might be life on Mars, that there were countless other planets, or that for a price, you could go to visit the moon and check it out for yourself? Even Vincent Van Gogh contemplated the stars and the heavens and that there is much more than we figured. My son says he was a redhead. That may explain it. We had a few redheads in our family. He was a homeless man with incredible talent. He believed in himself, he never received validation during his life. He saw the starry night. He painted it. No one understood him. I always knew he was different. Every brush stroke conveyed a landscape. He was a genius! Every stoke was a painting in itself. Van Gogh was the Shakespeare of painting. All the world will herald him who study him. The painting of his I appreciate the most is of the stars. Every brush stroke is individual. He was a conduit. He could join one person to another. He signed it, Vincent. He was a loser as the world perceived him. He is the best artist of all time.

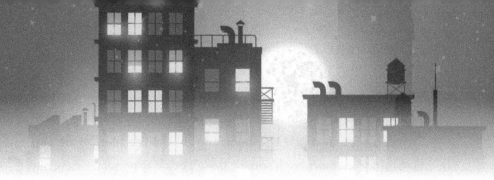

KEEPING IN TOUCH

As I turned on my radio and sat down to breakfast this morning, I realized it was Valentine's Day—the day of love . . . the day of hugs and kisses, of hearts and affection. Well, that's an exaggeration in this year of COVID. To find someone to wave at would be a nice treat. How we have had to stray this past year. It can be pretty lonely, especially on Valentine's Day. Friends no longer can come to call. Young people can no longer go skating or to prom or even out on a date. We've had to stay away from stores and stay away from parks where there are people. Stay away from the bank if you can manage it. Learn new ways of transferring money. Become a member of the cashless society . . . but that doesn't mean you can run up your Visa or Mastercard without repercussions, even if encouraged by your bank.

This Valentine's Day reminds me of one a long time ago when my husband and I went to visit my sister Ruby and husband, Jack. They invited us over to visit their friends in Silverdale. In departing, I gave the host a great big hug. He was so surprised and told me so. Actually, it was rather unusual for me, but Ruby hugs everybody and I just thought it was natural. I didn't know what to say, so I blurted out "Nobody gets too many hugs. Don't you agree?" We all had a good chuckle. In the days of COVID, the whole thing would be highly discouraged for fear of spreading the virus, but I'm sure everyone misses those kindly acts of friendliness—even the feel of a handshake or a simple touch. Think of the things we still can do to keep feelings alive in these trying times.

We can keep in touch by phone and on the Internet, so we can be thankful for that although some elderly people may not be clever in those regards. I had one friend who was really old-fashioned and was still being charged for every long-distance call she made rather than pay a little extra for long-distance by the month to anywhere she wanted. She wasn't short on money but had been brought up not spending an extra penny, so she sat at home waiting for everyone to call her.

Air travel is almost impossible unless you want to take the risk. You never know who would be contagious on the way or when you get there, relative or not. You may even take COVID with you. If you say, "Well you can always write letters," that's true. However, even getting them mailed can be a problem.

I almost forgot the Internet. The young people are fortunate, but we seniors may not be so savvy. The one you are messaging may not be geared up to respond at all.

We're discouraged from going to church meetings, and those who have ignored the caution have been punished by the worst kind of disease to strike even though you meant so well for yourselves and others, thinking you would be protected. COVID came from human actions and will be cured by all we can do with what God has given us.

March 2021

LOOKING BACK

On CBC—that's Canadian Broadcasting Company—they have some musicians presenting a program, and they're looking back on COVID, which wasn't recognized just a year ago. Now I look back and consider the lessons learned.

For me, it wasn't too hard to stay home day after day. I say that because I remember when I lived in Langley in my apartment. During that winter had the same feelings and I actually had to will myself to get out, go down to the parking garage, get the little car, go through the gate and just go somewhere. It was easier to stay in my comfortable surroundings, reading a book, catching up on office work and even writing in my journal.

I have thought during this year that I should remember growing up in Regina, Saskatchewan, when the days could drop to 40 below zero. I felt sorry for myself if I had to stay indoors no matter what weather. I would say to myself, "Get busy; don't feel sorry for yourself" an expression I got from my mother. She would sometimes let me go out, so I wouldn't annoy her by fighting with my little sister, Dorothy.

One of those times was when I convinced her to let me go ice skating. I hope I haven't told this story before. Anyway, I got my skates on not knowing how deathly cold it was out there and headed the block and a half to the outdoor skating rink. The streets and sidewalks were covered with ice and snow, so the trip was easy, as one could skate on the sidewalks and there wasn't a person in sight in that dark black frigid night. I felt rather cheerful upon arriving at the clubhouse shed, as the caretaker had built a big fire and he was puttering around, stirring up the coals for an empty audience. After a quick skate around the rink, I was ready to get warm and head off home. It wasn't much fun with no one there. I wished I had worn warmer mittens and heavier socks and a better scarf around my head, as it was sure cold. I started home. It was colder and colder, but I pushed on just about crying from the cold on my ears, fingers and toes.

Mother had little sympathy for me going skating on a night like that, but she helped me take off my skates, my coat, and leggings. She rubbed my ears to make the freezing go away and made me some hot chocolate. I vowed I would never do that again. Looking back, that was one cold, hard winter! I was glad when it was spring.

FIGHTING LONELINESS
DURING COVID

Looking around me, there are many things I could do to overcome being hemmed in here at home with no car and a dental appointment in two hours: I could sit and sulk. That's a no. I could clean the house. My husband, Charlie, used to tell people, "Belle works for eight hours cleaning the house and eight hours messing it up. I guess that's still true, but I have no intention to do too much today. I took care of the necessities yesterday. I could put on my mask and go for a walk. The few times I succeeded, it was amazing how other masked folks would cross the road without coming close to me, the other masked bandits. We're all loosening up now that we've had our shots, but I imagine that we're not too trusting because we don't know who has had their shots and who has refused them.

I could sit and mourn my dear friend's death. Ann had been sick for a long time. She was blind and probably had other complications in her old age. I hope she didn't have COVID. As far as I know, there was no funeral. Funerals as we know them are no more because we could be a semblance to the plague. My son Douglas suggested I write my obituary. At ninety-one, maybe I should, but it wasn't exactly something to cheer me up. He and his wife have done theirs, or so he suggested on the telephone from Alberta. My one hope in life is that I don't outlive my children . . . and there is a slight possibility as they are seniors themselves.

I have found the television a great comfort, and watching it is a great way to fall asleep in the chair. I bought a sixty-inch screen years ago. It was love at first sight. I find I watch publicly-owned stations like Knowledge Network here in Vancouver and KCTS9 in Seattle. Their historically based programs are wonderful. I wish my history teacher in high school was here to see how it's done. Oh, how we all hated memorizing dates and learning to spell Latin names. They both had too many to learn to pass the exams. The children of today learn so much more today from the wonderful programs they have.

I also watch the news channels including CHEK TV from Victoria. They have wonderful advertising too, but I'm not tempted, as it's a ferry ride away. However, if they only knew it, they could probably have more online sales. They're attractive even when you can't afford them.

With all that's happening, I find myself glued to the international news channels at certain hours, especially the nightly broadcast from the BBC, London, though I have Seattle's station on. *The View* is important to us in Vancouver although their news seems to stop at the forty-ninth Parallel. Come to think of it, they sometimes have a little news about Alaska but not often. I remember the earthquake of '64, mainly because we were on Vancouver Island that weekend and they were in for a tsunami, which hit the western side of the island.

We have little news about the Yukon. It has to be tragic to hit the airwaves. Los Angeles has their own stations, so that, too, is illuminated. Of course, in 2020, the terrible fires down there were seen across the world, as they were the worst in history. We didn't hear much about the Far East, which we know is in dire straights with millions of people being killed, and of course natural disasters around the world, one after another—not to mention global warming literally at our doorstep (we know they used to ice skate in New Westminster on the Fraser River here in the Lower Mainland at the turn of the twentieth century).

I still get letters from numerous charities for money for worthy causes. I can't say that cheers me up. I want to help them all, but with paying for my new roof I definitely have to postpone most, no matter how worthy they are. I often wonder why I'm on their list at all. I have given up my car, which sits in the lane immovable, not because of its cost but mainly because of my age. It has changed my life, but I do feel good about helping myself and helping the planet.

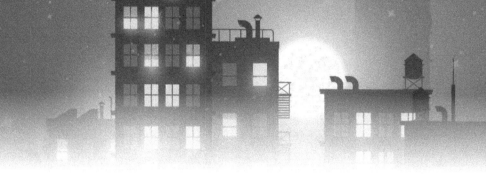

SOCIAL DISTANCING

Social distancing were two words I had never heard together a year ago. The grocery store I shop at didn't have the sign up telling us to line up, and they didn't have footprints to tell us which way to go or arrows pointing in the direction we're to walk. Oh yes, and that we are to wear masks. Mothers of twins complain about how much trouble the "pandemic parenting" is. I'm sure it is. Would it cheer them up if I mentioned how inconvenient it would be without pampers? Maybe not. Maybe if I told them that we had made the baby's diapers out of flannelette and had to wash them almost every day. Okay, so I have to admit that I wasn't long before I saved up for a wringer washing machine but we had no dryer except the sunshine on the clothesline. Did I hear, "Oh weird . . . and wonderful." Did the thoughts cheer you up about the life you have today, young mothers? I hope so.

Yes, having twins is twice the work. I agree. We had twins in our family. People ask, "Can you tell them apart?" I would answer, "Yes it's easy. One is a boy and one is a girl."

In case the term "social distancing" is new to you too, it means staying two meters apart in Canada and six feet apparat in the United States. Take your choice.

April 4, 2021

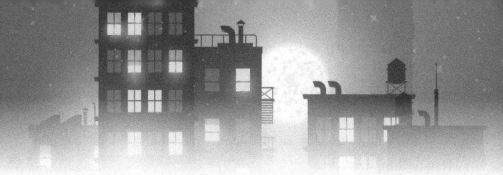

I WILL TAKE THE CHALLENGE
THAT MAKES ME HAPPY

FIVE THINGS THAT I AM GOOD AT

1. Writing. I love to write. It is the first thing that came to mind. Hope everyone agrees that I'm good at it.

2. Making hot chocolate. Don't laugh unless you've tried it.

3. Buying real estate. Notice I said "buying" not "selling."

4. Relating to people.

5. Being a grandmother, and a great grandmother and a great great grandmother. Shall I go on?

It's all amazing! It's what's missing that surprises me. I think of other people's accomplishments. Now, *that's* a list! I won't list them here, as the list could go on forever, but maybe I would start with Bill Gates. I think he's my hero. I used to carry a little picture as an example around with me in my day planner and I would tell people he went to the University of British Columbia, the same university my son went to and I really believed he did—until, of course, I found out the truth. He isn't even Canadian! He just changed the world. That's pretty good.

You will notice that my list doesn't mention that I was good at certain things:

1. Getting a college degree? Nope, but I went back to university at ninety years old and loved it.

2. An excellent cook? Nope.

3. A good speller? Nope, but I'm pleased Bill Gates gave me Spellcheck, even in Canadian, which no one seems to agree on.

4. A fine musician Nope? but I'm a good listener.

5. An actress on demand? Hardly. Especially not one of those with hardly any clothes on.

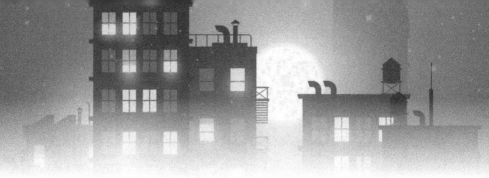

BLACK SKIN MATTERS

The Murder of George Floyd

The murder of George Floyd was one of the worst things I had the misfortune of witnessing. This police officer was placing his boot on the neck of George Floyd while another officer was just standing there looking on. George was crying out "I can't breathe, I can't breathe." If anything, the officer tightened down tighter and tighter as if to say, "Shut up, you _____. I'll show you."

I sat there unable to do anything, wondering if anyone would help him. There were people standing on the curb but the camera showed the look on the officer's face, daring them to move. Unshed tears filled my eyes knowing that I must help him but was unable to help from more than a thousand miles away. Even if I had been there, I wonder if I could have combatted the police without a weapon. My absolute admiration goes for whoever filmed the incident. They showed everything, including the other officer standing there watching the whole thing go on, and I do use the word in the biblical sense. I noticed the following day on some of the channels the news facts they had on the news that they had shortened or shall I say edited the tape to suit their perspective. I saw some of the court case as well, so I hope they don't do likewise.

I see the whole thing differently. I'd like to rewrite it all from the beginning if we could start all over again. I'm an author, so this is the way I wished the whole scenario had unfolded: The store owner may be Black or White. We'll call George, "Geo" He goes into the shop to buy whatever it was he needed. We'll call the store owner Mr. Mike. And the helper, Henry. Mr. Mike is behind the counter at the time. The helper is filling shelves.

George comes in and makes a purchase and produces a $20.00 bill. Mike is no dummy. He notices the bill doesn't look exactly right. He thinks it might be a counterfeit. In fact, he's almost sure it's a phony. He turns to the customer, who's a regular in there, and says, "I know you. Here's the bill back but keep what you purchased. Next time you come in, you can pay."

Geo. Says "Thanks, I appreciate that. I need it for the wife." He nods and goes out the door.

A friendship is made. Mr. Mike doesn't need to call the police. They are never involved when it's a suspected phony bill—especially for $20.00. He knows the police in the area. Drugs aren't an issue. He isn't drunk nor does he look dangerous. He's never brought in a counterfeit bill before. The boy loading the shelves can get on with his work. Maybe before the end of the trials, this may all become clear but it looks like the defense lawyer is trying to skip all this and the almost all-White jury will be on the side of the police and the store owner. Maybe the storekeeper was the one who was drunk.

The public will be ignored. The officers on duty will be found to be just doing their duty. It will be determined that killing another black man is insignificant. Business as usual. Nothing has changed. In fact, there have been more murders since, even at the time, Donald Trump encouraged his followers to cause as much mayhem as possible at the Capitol Building. The details will come out. The mentality was assessed. There has to be accountability to protect all of God's children, Red, White, Black, Grey, Brown or Blonde like me. It won't bring back George, but it will make it a better world.

I wonder if that policeman or any of the other police that were around that night realize today how stupid they were to allow another to kill their man for no reason.

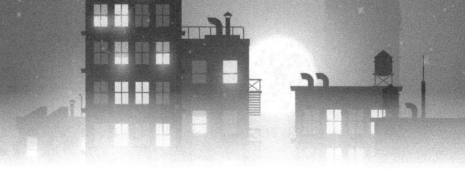

LOOKING TOWARDS
TOMORROW

1. I think of track star Roger Bannister, the winner of the four-minute mile, not because it happened right here in Vancouver but because they said it was impossible and he did it anyway. Now at the Olympics, they do it as a matter of course. They said at the Boston Marathon that anyone over thirty-nine couldn't possibly run 26.2 miles, but eventually, they did it anyway. They wouldn't let ladies run the Boston Marathon, but they eventually squeezed in and did it anyway. Let your motto be "I'll do it anyway." Now I don't mean to disobey orders but think of Roger Bannister and "do it anyway" even if someone says "it can't be done."

2. Never give up. There was a downturn in the economy not too long ago. "There are no jobs out there." Some people didn't believe them, and up popped Silicon Valley. I knew one of those young fellows. He just kept learning and trying. He's a multimillionaire today.

3. Empower others. That is a wonderful gift to have and to give. You will be well rewarded.

4. Don't be hindered by age. If you do, you may end up with Alzheimer's. My short-term memory was starting to go. It was frightening. I had always written journals and stories, but I've kept on going. I taught "Writing Your Family History" for twenty-five years, and people loved me for it. "Now that there is COVID, I can sit down and do nothing or I can press forward." That's what I told myself. I now write almost every day, and my mind has improved. It seems unbelievable! My spelling is still poor, but let's face it: there's still Spellcheck. And what I can do you can do double.

5. Read, read, read worthy literature, not nonsense, and you will amaze yourself. I read a few books a week if I can and have my one-and-only helper trot back and forth to the library for me to pick up the volumes I need, and she browses the Internet to find what I need to order.

6. Write, write, write. Set a time if possible.

7. Exercise. Set a time. Enjoy what you're doing.

8. Make your own list and follow it. My time is short and so is yours.

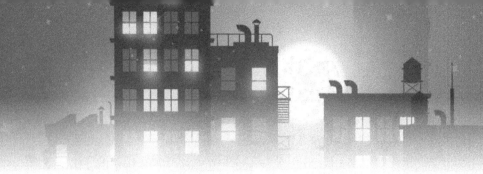

THE HEATWAVE OF '21

I t isn't enough to have COVID around the world but we have just come through the first day of a heatwave like none other that's ever happened. Many cities in Canada are hotter than Vegas. I may be wrong, but 48°C seemed to be rattled around on the news and that's on the Richter scale of course. There have been many emergencies concerning elderly people and as many as twenty-five deaths, but don't quote me; it might be larger. People have phoned into 911 (that's 999 in Britain) and had to stay on the line, an unheard-of thing until it was too late, then wait for an ambulance, wondering what was holding them up, the poor darlings.

I was trying to follow the rules to stay cool, stay home or under the trees. I'm sure they thought everyone had air conditioning. Sorry, less than 25 percent have air conditioning here in British Columbia. I remember in Palm Springs, they were used to the heat and had a saying that when the heat reached 100 or more, they would stay home under the air conditioning or in the car with the air conditioning running or in a shopping mall. Yes, this is Southern BC, but that is rather a misnomer

I, for one, am luckier than most, in a way, as I have an air conditioner of sorts that a tradesman sold to me second-hand a couple of years ago when there was a hot period in August. He also set it up in the window in the bedroom. It worked handsomely during that short period, but

I found it rather expensive. As long as I stayed in that section of the house, I was glad I had it. The opposite is true in the living room during the winter. I keep the fireplace going. Small fans help in the summer. My office was like a furnace that year, as it's in the sunroom. That year, I came very close to succumbing to the extreme heat.

I decided I would have to be creative, so on Monday, I put in a load of wash in cold water, which I always do, as the washer has no hot water setting—no hot water pipe actually. Then, I took it out, and instead of drying the clothes outside in that heat and certainly not in the dryer downstairs, I plunked it down, helter-skelter on the chesterfield blanket in the living room, hoping that would help bring down the temperature. I think it did, too. I'll swear it dried in two hours. Then, it was hot as usual. I was spinning. My head was spinning. The news on the television reported deaths and a shortage of hospital beds.

Come suppertime, there was no way I was going to light the electric stove and boil, roast, microwave, toast, fry, or cook anything, but I managed. Teemy, the gal downstairs, brought home two litre-sized chocolate milks, so with a bit of skim added, I managed quite well. I'm gaining weight during COVID because of lack of exercise anyway.

Besides, I had eaten all the treats in the cupboard weeks ago. I'm fond of almonds (with chocolate on top of course). I know they are good for me, but I'm not so sure about the chocolate.

Time for bed. It was so hot in the bedroom, I knew I could never sleep. I had washed another load of clothes, taken two showers that day (which helped a little), and decided I would strip down the bed and myself and put a wet towel on the mattress cover. I felt the mattress might be marked, but my life would be saved, so it was worth it. This was all before I figured out to connect that hand-me-down air conditioner.

I actually slept very well.

The next morning, the sun came streaming through the window. I thought I knew what hot was, having lived on the prairies the first seventeen years of my life, but nothing like this. I was born in Brandon, Manitoba, under rather unusual circumstances, which I mention in *Finding My Family*, but why my mother had gone there I do not know, and the most of my youth, I lived in Regina, Saskatchewan. We never were in a position to own an air conditioner- never knew what one was—but almost everyone was in the same circumstances. I had taken this new purchase out of the window for the winter so as to refrain from letting the winter breezes come in, and there it lay all crumpled on the floor—no connection in sight—and it was too hot to beat it into submission. Besides that, it was the day for my second COVID vaccination, wouldn't you know? How was I going to survive?

I looked for cool clothing. It was exasperating! I found a swimsuit in a drawer. I wiggled into it but it was too tight. Tried another. Same verdict. Found a swim top but couldn't find the bottom. It had a built-in bra, so I put it on, followed by a pair of shorts, which I swear no one had ever seen me wear. It would have to do. A wet tea towel completed the ensemble. I was sure others would be wearing rather original thrown-together clothing as well. Five, maybe six people died within a few days from the heat. I'm fortunate to be here, and I know it. It was close. I had never come so close to succumbing to that dreadful heat.

My life was at stake at the senior centre in Kerrisdale, where they were waiting to vaccinate me. The appointed time was at 4:15, the hottest time of the afternoon. It wasn't the quick poke of the needle that I feared but dying of "temperature overdose," a new name for sunstroke.

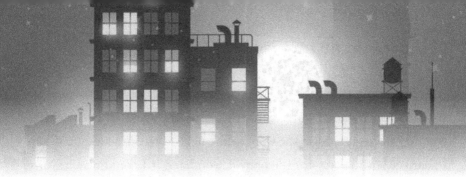

GLOBAL WARMING

The next day, the heat went on. My mother would say, "Not a breath of air filled the atmosphere." I kept thinking to myself, *I hope people start being attentive and do something about global warming. Talk is cheap but it can't help get us active in global warming. This heat is killing me.*

The trip to Kerrisdale to get my second antibody shot went well, although Themi's car doesn't have air conditioning. She found parking about a block away, and the street did have shade under the trees. She let me off and walked from there to the entrance to the senior centre which I appreciated. One thing that was on my mind was the high number of deaths these past few days. They haven't been from COVID but, rather, the heat waves . . . especially old folks like me and the fact people can't get an answer to their 911 calls and are put on hold for long periods plus waiting for an ambulance that is trying its best to reach all the patients. What will happen in a worse disaster? A young mother of a two-month-old was one of the people waiting and it was a really dangerous situation. We only heard of it because it was on CBC.

Mothers are often not very old themselves. They're not used to the responsibility of the cute little creature God has blessed them with and may not have all the talk this young woman gave but I did hear that they didn't have air conditioning, which is common, so what did she do? I couldn't imagine.

She took the baby in the car and went looking for an air conditioner. When she arrived at the store, they had all been sold as you may have guessed so she went to the next store. Same result. When I heard. I felt so sorry for the baby. I wondered if I could give her any advice that would have helped. I'm no expert, but I can tell you what I have learned recently. It may help. Number 1: the modern way seems to be is to use the Internet to see if they have any in stock and if they can deliver or you have to pick it up. It's so dangerous to take a child in a hot car and worse to leave him or her there even for a few minutes in front of a building—or anywhere really. Children and pets die in cars every year because they have been left.

I like to buy locally, but more and more businesses are on the net as well as having a shop. Yes, sometimes you have to pay for delivery, but most of the time, there are ways around it.

Not every mother could even afford to shop for any extras and in that case, I would suggest you keep the baby at home and let him or her bathe in a cool tub or a basin like Grandma used to do. Older children would be so happy with a paddling pool but these must be well supervised. It could be fun for the whole family. Wet towels are also good to cool down the children and yourselves, even a washcloth. The water hose is great fun as well. It does double duty.

Everyone knows that this planet's warming has been evident for a long time and this is only going to continue. In my own life, I have seen the glaciers shrink, and the winters get warmer. Moreover, the Fraser River near Cloverdale where we used to skate no longer freezes over. I've seen all that man has done to hasten our demise. If there is something you can make or someone you can help with education so they can make the world better, you too will be rewarded.

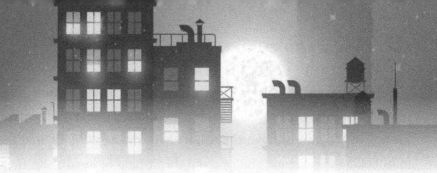

THE MYSTERY OF THE TWO PUSSY CATS

Do you have any pets at home?" asked the denturist as she peered into my mouth with a long sharp instrument.

"No, I mumbled," but the lady living upstairs has a big dog and a cat.

"Oh, I guess that's enough for one house."

"Yes, I like it when the cat comes down for a visit. Do you have a cat?"

"No, but I have a little dog. That keeps me busy."

"Why do you ask?"

"Well, the funniest thing happened at our house recently. We heard a meowing in the garage. It's an old garage, and there's an opening where this mother cat and her baby kitten were found curled up in the corner on a pile of cardboard. We were very surprised to see them and wondered if they were hungry, so we brought out some milk and some of our dog's food.

"At first, they were very timid, so we just left it there and came back the next morning. The food was all gone, so we brought out more food, and we wondered if they were friendly and if we could pet them. The mother was very happy when we patted and cuddled her, but the kitten stayed close to its mother.

"We wondered where they came from. They became more friendly almost right away, and, soon they allowed us to take them into the house. We searched, but they didn't have any tags. We figured they must belong to someone, though, and they would be looking for them. Our children asked if we could keep them. 'Please?' said Timmy, our youngest.

'They're so pretty,' said Patty our oldest. 'Can I have the mother? I love her grey fur and her white paws.'

'If we don't find the owners, we can all share, and that means we all have to look after them. I've put an ad in the paper and nailed a lost-and-found poster on the telephone pole. Maybe our neighbours down at the corner will recognize them. Your father has certainly grown attached to them; he'll miss them if we find the owners. See how he lets them cuddle up to him while he is watching television? And see how the little one is growing?'

'Can we give them names?'

'Yes, you can name them, but remember they may belong to someone else.'

'Well, seeing that it's during COVID,' interrupted Dad, 'Let's call the mother Covy and the baby...'

'And the baby?' came a voice from the chair. 'Let's just call it Kitty.'

'Sounds good to me. It's decided for now.'

We were all a happy family until, one day, I decided to put a little sign up on the telephone pole on the corner asking if anyone had lost a cat. As the little kitten whom they called Kitty grew bigger and our dog, Ginger, just didn't get along and often the living room would end up a mess of papers all over the place.

Then, it was decided that we would put another sign up on another telephone pole where the children passed to go to school.

Sure enough, a day or two later, the telephone rang, and the lady on the other end of the line said that they had lost a cat with grey fur and two white paws. She came over, and Covy ran over to her and jumped into her arms. It was a happy reunion. It was her cat. They did belong to that family. The mother cat had probably wanted to get away by herself to have her kitten, as her owners had a large family and cats are very wise. Now they were reunited and live happily ever after.

You may wonder why I put this story in this COVID book. I wonder myself. Let's say "for comic relief." It's been a hard two years, and some may need the break.

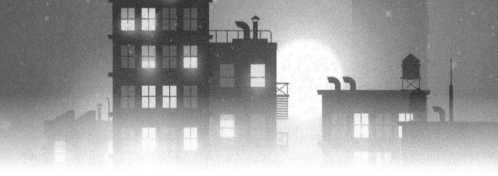

SLOGANS

D r. Bonnie Henry, Health Minister had a slogan for everyone: "Be kind, be calm, be safe. She was well-respected, and she was gifted a necklace, which she came to be known for wearing every broadcast, which was every day. She set the example and those who followed her advice were rewarded.

PIONEERS AND THEIR HEALTH AND DISEASES

At the time of the Saskatchewan pioneers, there were few medical aids, so it's important to see how the first settlers managed to live on the prairies. I'll go back to 1912 when the Smiths arrived at their homestead in Riverhurst on the River Saskatchewan, approximately seventy-nine miles from Moose Jaw. Each family was given forty acres of land and was charged $10.00. They were given so many years to clear the land, build a home, and plant wheat on the farm. My mother would have been seventeen years old when they arrived with her parents, the Smiths, her sister Minni, who was nine years older than my mother-to-be, and Minni's husband, Mel Anderson. In 1913, Mabel, my mother, married Chester Ray, who worked on the ferry, which ran from the Riverhurst side to the Meadow Lake side, the west side of the Saskatchewan River. There were no doctors in the area at first, so when someone got sick or had babies, the mother had the baby at home or they had to go as far as Moose Jaw to the hospital. Of course, there was no medical coverage, so it was costly to go to a hospital. Most babies were born at home with the help of a neighbour if they were lucky. Chester's mother, Dora Ray, helped give birth to many children in those sod huts that the pioneers had built.

Imagine the cold, below zero winters with the river frozen over and how difficult it would be. My oldest brothers and sisters were born there, and my brother Fred died at birth or when he was very young and is buried out there on the prairie. I'm sure my mother was devastated.

Eventually, there was one doctor for the whole district, and he would make his rounds with his horse and buggy to all the farmers and their families. It may sound romantic, but somehow, I doubt it.

I'm sure he would be busy with the settlers having accidents on farm machinery, falling on the ice, being kicked by a cow, falling off a horse or a ladder. The list goes on. The Smiths and the Andersons with their first daughter gave up homesteading and went back to Minnesota in 1918 but Alex's brother "Doc" stayed behind. Unfortunately, he fell on the icy steps at the ferry and broke his chin. He refused any attention at first, but as time passed, it became clear that it was serious, and Chester took him all the way to Moose Jaw to the hospital, where he died. We're not sure if it was because of his injury or the Spanish flu, which was rampant at that time all around the world. I'm sure mother was deeply grieved as he had helped raise her along with the Smiths ever since they got her when she was three years old. It was a sad story.

Many pioneers lost their lives in similar ways. When the ice broke in the spring, many a sled (complete with the horses, gear and driver) went floating down the river. Uncle Ed Ray was one of them. Fortunately, he was saved, but the rest was lost. Finally, Mel, Minnie, and their daughter went back to Minnesota in 1918 just in time for World War I, although I don't think they were involved. Grandpa Alex Smith and Grandma Jessie accompanied them. Grandpa still had his cows, and I never heard if he finally accepted pasteurization or not. Mother never talked about them with us, but we studied about Madam Curie in school.

I didn't mention sicknesses among the pioneers, but they were numerous. The common cold could result in pneumonia, which could lead to death. Colds were contagious. There were no inoculations, vaccinations, or anything else that we take for granted today. Here are some of the choices the pioneers had. I don't recommend any of the old remedies, but we do use some of them today. Nothing has been found to cure COVID, as it's a virus and destroys all in its path.

1. Liquor – I grew up in a liquor-free home, so I wouldn't recommend it for anything, but I'm sure it was a good excuse to cure some disease that came along—especially for the man of the house.

2. Baking soda and water – I think mother used that so we wouldn't scratch our mosquito bites or measles. Perhaps it works.

3. Chicken soup – That was deemed to cure everything, and I'm sure it was great comfort food. They may have added rice and vegetables to it. Barley soup was also popular.

4. Compresses – These were used for open wounds, sores, and all sorts of things. Comprised mainly of rags.

5. Early to bed and early to rise – Just being sent to bed was known to help or, let's say, "Time was on their side." It worked for depression. It certainly helped bring about good health (or so it seemed).

6. Mother's stew with vegetables – Yes, good nutrition was important, but poverty was common.

7. Carter's Little Liver Pills — I don't know if they ever worked for anything, but they were popular.

8. And there was the Watkin's man, who went door-to-door around the prairies with his wares. My older siblings tell of their father being jealous of Mother and the Watkins man and the fight that ensued as she said how silly he was for even thinking that. He did sell such things as cod liver oil, and I remember having to swallow a tablespoon of it every morning during the winter. It was quite a fighting match to watch.

9. Later, I remember Mother buying vanilla from a Watkins man. (Not the same one, I'm sure.) He swore it to be the real thing—the real vanilla. I doubt very much her "entertaining" him with a house full of kids at her heels. He was very important to the settlers, though, as it was extremely difficult to go to a grocery store, which was miles away.

10. Low blood flow — I don't know if they knew anything about that, but settlers got lots of exercise, so few lived long enough to get Alzheimer's.

11. Inflammation — This was something the settlers talked about, but I don't know if they had a cure.

12. Sugar wasn't a problem as it is today, as it was mainly found in natural foods and proved expensive. Fruits weren't available, although I remember rhubarb and picking chokecherries and saskatoons to make jam. I have rhubarb in the yard today. Cakes also had sugar.

13. Head injury from running with the bulls – They may have had injury through falls, but I think the first idea was uncommon. Maybe modern "settlers" don't want to get a vaccination because of some brain injury for that reason. I sometimes wonder what they are suffering from.

15. It wasn't usual for them to have fresh fruit, but at Christmas, we usually had a box of Satsuma oranges from Japan. We called them Japanese oranges and loved them. Thirty years later, the doctor would tell you that you only had to eat one orange a day to get all the vitamin C that you need. I don't know what he would say today. Maybe the same but we know a lot more about vitamins now than they did then, and we're learning more every year. It would be wonderful if there was one to cure COVID.

16. Cinnamon – This was a common spice used by early settlers, but they probably didn't know it was good for them. They just knew it tasted good.

TRIALS OF THE PIONEERS

The prairies as I remember them once you got out of the big city of Regina at about 84,000 people it was just one long railway track from west to east called the CPR. Of course, there was the CNR as well, but as children, we never considered it part of our lives, nor did we consider ourselves pioneers. Our parents were the pioneers and they would tell us about the hard days they had health-wise, which I would like to relate to you to prepare you for the future after COVID (and to deal with the present moment). Health, of course, was important to pioneers, and they had many problems and many diseases to contend with. Among them were fever and the flu—and head and chest colds were commonplace as they are today. More serious though, was tonsilitis which I had in my teenage years and had to have my tonsils out. There was strep throat, jaundice, asthma lumbago, pleurisy, inflammatory rheumatism and quinsy, infectious eye diseases, pink eye trachoma, and many others that I even can't remember. Then, there were the contagious diseases that I may have mentioned before like tuberculosis, diphtheria, whooping cough, measles, mumps, chickenpox, smallpox, typhoid, and scarlet fever. The list is long, and they transferred from one family to another without question of who was to get it next. It was only with the introduction of inoculations that there was any let-up. We today are so fortunate. I suppose there are people around who think that they just disappeared. That's not true.

In fact, even those who are still on the earth could break out and multiply as it did in 1902 when an epidemic of diphtheria broke out, which fortunately my mother lived through. Many people did not. Thousands died, many of them children. My mother would have been twelve years old. Some pioneers at that time feared inoculations and just wouldn't accept them. Pity.

Some settlers blamed bad river water for all their troubles (and they were partly right) or they blamed old wells for having bad water. Everyone had their own theory—sometimes correct, sometimes not. Sometimes the cow's milk was blamed or something they ate. Sometimes misdiagnosis happened, and the treatment for the disease didn't work because it wasn't that at all. Many died because of the lack of getting any help at all. Doctors and nurses were scarce, and often, the settlers had no money for care. It wasn't until the 1950s that we had any public medical care. Quarantine usually meant the mother staying home with the children and the husband not being allowed in the house until the quarantine was lifted by the health inspector. He would probably go to the house of a neighbour or his parents and bring food for the family and put it over the fence. A sign would be put on the door or the fence that said "Quarantined" to protect any would-be visitors. It was important to keep those who were sick away from other members of the family.

We still have a long way to go, as the saying goes, but with the science laboratories, we have today we should be thankful and take advantage of the myriad of advancements we have made. We will need more scientists, doctors and nurses, though. Education will probably be everyone's greatest achievement.

COVID times may slow many down but not defeat them if you agree the few simple rules. Vaccination may be the greatest gift you will receive. This pandemic will attack everyone if given the chance—rich and poor, the good and the bad, the faithful and those who have never seen the inside of a church or temple—no matter what someone else thinks. Everyone has freedom of choice. However, in making the wrong choice, you endanger those around you—especially those you love. In breaking the rules, you also put the nurses and doctors and caregivers at risk and as my mother would say, "They won't be there when you need them." Every day they put themselves at risk to save those who can't be bothered.

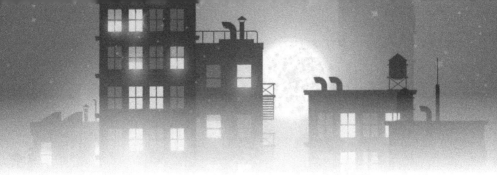

COVID AFTERMATH

So far, I haven't gotten any reports on whether there is any aftermath to COVID or are we left to wonder "When we get a cough or a cold is it COVID and if I had COVID, is it coming back?" Of course, because I haven't had it once I shouldn't worry about the after-effects, but I do. Truthfully, I only hear that someone is in the hospital or that they have passed away. However, I have put out feelers and maybe someone who writes in will tell us how everything is affecting them.

*   *   *

Our four granddaughter's stepdad passed away with COVID. So many people are finding they have a family now with the DNA processes.

We are very boring and don't go anywhere anymore. Point Roberts is really hurting from lack of business due to COVID. We are seeing shortages.

Love Marlene York

Oct 15, 2021

*   *   *

Hi Belle,

Here is a pandemic story for you.

My granddaughter Belle was married a few weeks ago in the Portland temple, and we really wanted to attend. The land border was closed, so we couldn't drive down to Portland.

We didn't feel comfortable flying even though we've been fully vaccinated. I have to be especially cautious because I'm still on dialysis. So yes, the COVID restrictions have caused some frustration for our family. John and his family will be coming for a visit in November, thank goodness. We haven't seen them for two years, and his newest daughter Giovanna is almost two; it will be so good to meet her at last!

I'm scheduled to have a booster shot next week, which I'm happy about!

Love,
Yvonne♥♥♥
October 10, 2021

*   *   *

For me: "the COVID-19 Pandemic" served as a springboard and catalyst for "self-inquiry" in all of its many manifestations.

"What do I really stand for?" (For example) . . . "Who am I REALLY?

Can "WHO I REALLY am" be affected by life's apparent storms? In other words; the "TRUTH" . . . setting us free . . . ?

Free to? Free to: "re-invent ourselves and our agendas"?

Free to allow playfulness, creativity, spontaneity, and "connection" . . . to run our lives?

I discovered a lot about myself.

Besides an innate curiosity, I'd been blessed with resilience and resourceful thinking.

The belief "that I was/would be forever supported by the Universe/"withstanding the tests of time . . ."

I prevailed (and . . . "AND HOW!!!").

The writing process definitely carried me through the challenging times! Writing and painting "connected me to myself," ushering forth the playful, artistic and clever "inner-me!"

The pandemic taught me to be more "present" and accountable for "this precious time here on Earth."

Hetty Willeumier is a long-time aficionado of good literature; revealing life's many customs and adventures etc.! Besides her love of reading, she enjoys writing, watercolour painting, and creating little characters in expressive gestures!

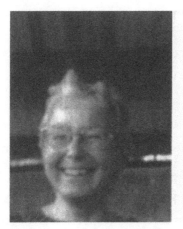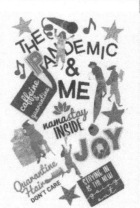

Art made by Hetty Willeumier

*   *   *

Alone and Together
by Cynthia Sharp

I open to sky clouds and blue summer yield to the peace of lying still back eases into alignment injuries subside this life I wish I'd shared with you I surrender to solitude creation and writing focus lying in wild daisies like I did in my twenties, wishing you were with me that we hadn't been cut apart.

It's the kind of July day when mellow music drifts in windows over neighbours watering lawns. You could almost forget there's a pandemic in Vancouver a break between bouts of wildfire smoke, water shortages and heatwaves, for a few days or weeks, an almost normalcy.

Sounds of peace open time mallards' quiet cypress in wind gardening reading the hail of uninterrupted leisure of choice I keep going back to the window, a calm, safe life beyond these walls, mild adventure, connection.

I dance dreams into plays, existence a learning curve, starting and ending on gratitude.

When the sky cools, I look to the sunscapes the glass jars on the counter create on the wall, each one different, catching the light in a unique way, the black cherry jar a mirage of diamonds, now a hummingbird angel.

It's one of those days when the clouds break up into millions, an explosion of atoms into the universe, and we lay orange lilies on lawns, a tribute to heroes on the front lines.

I ask myself who I want to go through the pandemic with and answer community members with vision, respect, and depth. Real work . . .

Five-hour meditation is perfect for my back. Rest, rest, rest. Then, yoga—the relief of accomplishment, an explosion of bright colour, living spirit, oxygen released like worlds bursting forth, my breath the sails propelling me along an ocean let me be longer at peace . . . hope like islands of grass in the sun

What to do with my perfectly restored meditative energy learning to keep wellness for health and service to let go?

I forget everything else I had wanted to say—just gratitude for real community and purpose. Not because there's anything more than this life but because I value a culture of meaning and kindness. Just by being in the world, you've taught me so much about self-acceptance and love. We stretch like July trees, realizing we've grown.

The lightness of free time, voices cycling past my window in the summer evening, the signal of permission, children's calls, the freedom of not having to be anywhere, the return of time.

We're all ordinary these days and there's something beautiful in that, our regular un-styled hair and selves. Accede, bow, stay home, stay safe, let the eagles carry our dreams.

* * *

Even If These Are Our Last Days
by Cynthia Sharp

Even if the virus takes us this season
I still want to be present
to this gently unfolding
middle day of the week
to spring poetry
sounds and smells of ordinary

the normalcy of Byron across the street
playfully shovelling top soil in his garden
to fertilize summer crops
the possibility that it's okay
permission to live simply
to enjoy the wealth of books I have
Audre Lorde this afternoon
healing recovery breath
handling what we reasonably can
to cultivate deep meaning
with a small number of people
I just want this to be a normal Wednesday
in the sunlight with cherry trees
to curl up in bed with the partner
I'm still hoping for
and tell him everything I loved
about our life
clasp hands and remember
all the funny moments of our decades
knowing we are blessed
to have shared it all
coop handfuls of yellow split peas
and drop them slowly into a silver pot
to boil into carrot cabbage soup
with a dollop of real butter
and a sprinkle of Atlantic Sea salt
time for dishes the comfort of washing
grateful for electricity and running water
palms and wrists relaxing in the hot stream

with biodegradable fragrance-free soap
bubbling in the air
the right to calm to sabbatical
even if only a day a week a month
maternity leave for self-care
fewer atmospheric pollutants
this summer a break for the Earth
from the intensity of smog
simple pleasures
amid cherry blossoms

Cynthia Sharp is a fine arts graduate student inspired by the rainforests and Pacific shoreline of her west coast home. She's a full member of the League of Canadian Poets as well as The Writers' Union of Canada and was the City of Richmond, British Columbia's, 2019 Writer in Residence. Her work can be found in many journals including CV2, Pocket-Lint, Untethered, and The Pitkin Review and in her collection Rainforest in Russet.

Oct 13, 2021

*   *   *

MY DEDICATION TO SYNTHIA SHARP
BY BELLE CURD

NOVEMBER 6, 2021

Synthia, you will be so happy to know that a violet-throated hummingbird was sighted in our yard right here in Vancouver, B.C.

At this time of year. I dedicate the finding to you, having read your lovely poem.

You may not be so happy about the next event, but last night, we had a black-out in our area, not in the whole of the city. I was frightened as it was so unusual. We never have electric outages, so I was afraid it would last a long time: There were so many "what ifs."

What caused it? What if the fridge thawed? What if it lasted a long time—like a week? What emergency heat do we have? The thought crossed my mind that we had none. Zip!

"Forget it, Belle" came a voice from within.

"There is nothing you can do right now. Your blankets are warm. You have another bundled up someplace just in case. I think the furnace is on. If it is, it will stay on. If it's on 'off' at the moment, well... don't even think about it"

With that, I bundled up and went back to sleep. Four hours later, I heard what I thought was a *click*, the sound of the lights going on somewhere in the house.

Was it all a signal to be prepared? How incredible to live through the pandemic and face another catastrophe? Some of us never learn.

Love one another,
Belle

*　*　*

"Frustrating Puzzlement" by Cynthia Hadden (Oct. 24, 2021)

COVID. The word permeates our thoughts,

our actions. Confusing us all.

What to believe?

Masks hiding faces. Do I know that person,

maybe not? Say hello anyway.

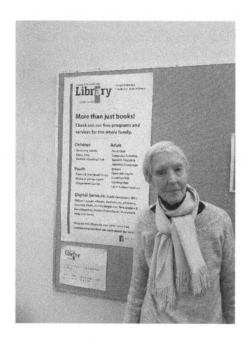

We do that in Gibsons.

Muffled voices unable to understand. Speak louder you ask.

Louder muffled voices.

Can't get too close. Double vaxxed? You dare not ask.

Sanitize hands then touch a doorknob. Clean? Maybe not.

You sanitize your hands again.

Hourly news reports numbers going up around the world,

vaccinations down.

Which province has the most COVID patients, most vaccinated?

Is this a competition?
Wear masks. Just inside? Just outside? Limit the numbers allowed.
Hundreds go to sports games.
The numbers of hospital patients rise. Nurses,
doctors plead for help while trying to
hold on.
What is open? Restaurants close. Small businesses go out of business
COVID becomes a seasonal illness like the flu.
The virus keeps mutating. Line up for
two vaccines.
So, we accept the new normal. Show your
QR code ID to get inside. Sit apart.
While theatres lose money from empty seats.
We are at war with viruses invisible to the
naked eye. We put on our boxing
gloves, build up our muscles. Ready to fight again.

*   *   *

I'm Afraid – A One-Act Play
By Del Lobo (Oct. 24, 2021)

JAKE: Is that a new skirt?

KASSIE: I bought it last year but never had the chance to wear it.

JAKE: Like the shirt I'm wearing. Mom sent it to me last Christmas, but who wears new clothes in front of a screen?

KASSIE: Is this the right platform?

JAKE: Yep, going in the right direction too.

KASSIE: I'm not sure I want to get on the train

JAKE: Why?

KASSIE: I'm afraid.

JAKE: Everyone is wearing a mask, and the train's almost empty.

KASSIE: Everyone?

JAKE: Okay, most then. We can avoid the ones who aren't wearing them.

KASSIE: I'm afraid.

JAKE: And I am friggin sick of it all.

KASSIE: You'll be sicker under a ventilator trying to catch your breath.

JAKE: We're missing opportunities.

KASSIE: I'm okay with *Zoom*.

JAKE: Yeah . . . but we need the energy of real people . . . real people, Kassie.

KASSIE: I can tell you're mad.

JAKE: How?

KASSIE: Because you called me Kassie and not Kas.

JAKE: I'm disappointed, okay? Restaurants are open, we're double-vaccinated. I'm hungry for people . . . what's that look?

KASSIE: Do I count as a person?

JAKE: Geez Kas, you know what I mean.

KASSIE: No, I'm not sure . . . how can it be that . . .

JAKE: There you go again with those unfinished sentences. For God's sake, say what you mean.

KASSIE: I mean you're being an ass.

JAKE: Oh! Because I crave connection with real people and want to talk face-to-face instead of on a screen, I'm an ass now?

KASSIE: Would it make you happier if I said you're a jerk instead?

JAKE: I think we should quit this now.

KASSIE: Okay boss, whatever you say.

JAKE: I don't like your tone.

KASSIE: Seems as if you don't like a lot about me.

JAKE: You know, I'm gonna agree with you. All this is making me angry.

KASSIE: Maybe your anger has nothing to do with me.

JAKE: Of course not. Who's being an ass now?

KASSIE: You've called me worse names before.

JAKE: Can we please . . . please . . . stop this?

JAKE: OMG! You're going to bring up old shit?

KASSIE: Why not? Let's take your anger up a notch.

JAKE: Sounds like you wanna fight. We could've avoided this by getting on the train.

KASSIE: You don't care that I'm afraid.

JAKE: I never said that. I'm just hoping that you get over it so that we can resume our life.

KASSIE: Did it ever occur to you that this might be life from now on?

JAKE: Sounds hopeless to me.

KASSIE: It is hopeless!

JAKE: I have an idea. Why don't we jump in front of the next train when it arrives?

KASSIE: Now you're being stupid.

JAKE: Am I? You're the one who said life is hopeless.

KASSIE: Here comes the train . . . hey, where are you going?

JAKE: I'm gonna go talk to that woman who just came in.

KASSIE: Maybe she needs help with her bags.

JAKE: Maybe she does.

KASSIE: Maybe you'll fall in love. It won't be the first time. Stop rolling your eyes. You know as well as I do that it's true. Don't you walk away while I'm . . . hey, look, she's not wearing a mask.

Del Lobo studies Creative Writing at the University of Guelph. Her work has appeared in Canadian Stories and an anthology titled "Constellations" She currently lives on the Sunshine Coast, B.C.

*   *   *

FINDING WAYS TO FEEL GOOD DURING COVID
BY: LAUREL SUKKAU / APRIL 2021

Does feeling good mean that we're not taking the situation seriously? Not at all. Feeling good is perhaps the best way to strengthen our immune system. Here are three of my favourite new pastimes.

Number one is online shopping. I love online shopping because this enjoyment unfolds in stages. First, there's the actual shopping. So fun! so fast! so easy! Perusing, selecting, and choosing. Then comes the thrill of anticipation until the delivery arrives. For me, this is usually one to three weeks, and by this time, I've often forgotten exactly what I've ordered, so I get to experience the joy all over again. Unboxing has become a sort of life metaphor as I look forward daily to some new surprising delight landing on my doorstep—a rare and precious insight, a never-before noticed snatch of birdsong, a beautiful new shade of pansy.

I've also found pleasure in gardening. Not serious gardening, more like throwing a few seeds in some dirt. But it is immensely satisfying to watch those little green sprigs popping up out of the bare ground after weeks of waiting. I'm surprised to be enjoying the waiting, the sense of allowing something to take its time. I suppose that's called patience.

My third therapeutic joy is baking—me and my little red hand mixer conjuring up a treat whenever the occasion calls for it. Recently, this was cupcakes with royal icing in marbled pastel hues. How enjoyable to watch the egg whites and sugar mixture pile up into glossy peaks and then add delicate swirls of food colouring. A treat for the eyes as well as the taste buds. It's been many years since I whipped up a batch of royal icing, it being on my forbidden foods list. How much fun to enjoy these little treats now and then. This is called living it up in lockdown.

I'm happy to share these examples with you and invite you to think about the everyday things that make you feel good, no matter what's happening in the world around you. Cheers!

Laurel Sukkau is a long-time resident of the Sunshine Coast, BC, and a member of the local Beachcombers Advanced Toastmasters Club. She is currently participating in a filming blog called Encompass.

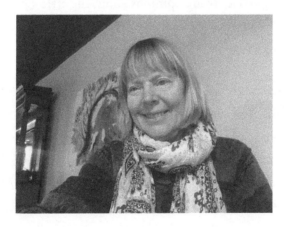

*   *   *

Having never had COVID, I don't have a personal story to share, but I can tell you that my wife, (a retired CRNP) and I are strongly anti-COVID vaccination!

Doctor Robert Malone, the developer of the messenger RNA technology that is being used in most of these vaccines, has grave reservations about MRNA being used as a COVID treatment. He believes the current vaccines available from Pfizer, Moderna, Johnson & Johnson (Jansen), and AstraZeneca are ineffective, poorly tested, and highly dangerous.

I do support the use of Ivermectin and Hydroxychloroquine with zinc as safe and effective treatments for the virus.

I've just had my second shingles vaccination and my wife gets her flu shots every year, so we aren't anti-vaccination . . . just anti-COVID vaccination.

You may have a different view, Belle, but as you can probably infer from the above, I have strong opinions about the efficacy of the current crop of COVID vaccines as well as about our highly politicized FDA and big pharma.

Author, Mike Sackett, has won numerous awards for his work, both as a writer and writing teacher. A past conference chairman of the Maryland Writers' Association, Mike's novel, The Striped Lion, won the MWA grand prize (and a publishing contract) as best novel in all genres. Jack Hanna wrote the book's foreword and Mike donated all his royalties to Jack's wildlife charity, Partners in Conservation, providing veterinary care to Rwanda's mountain gorilla.

The Face Painter, Mike's non-fiction short story about his years face-painting children in Johns Hopkins oncology wards, won first place in

MWA's yearly contest for best non-fiction short story. Retitled The Ride Home, an edited version of The Face Painter was published in Marlo Thomas & friends' New York Times best-seller, The Right Words at the Right Time – Volume II.

Mike's children's book, When Grandfather Sailed Away, which he also illustrated, was recently republished in India, in the Malayalam language.

*   *   *

Hmmm. Belle, I didn't write the piece you asked . . . but as there is a COVID-19 outbreak here in the Yukon, I feel I do want to share my views on the whole thing.

And climate change! ha-ha

I keep feeling that we should all take a step back, which truly is a step forward to peace and harmony—a good life or whatever else we might call it.

Many of us in society have reached a level (years ago for me and for me my whole life) that is full. We always have enough food, always have shelter, always have clean water . . . and what else? you get my point. From now on, it's only haul water and chop wood, or as Yukoners like to say chop water and haul wood.

So, let's do that. Let's each look into our own life where we can step back. If we all make choices that work for us, we won't have a COVID problem, which to me we don't have anyway. Like when I get sick, I draw within and look after myself in ways that work for me.

Hmmm, so what did I do today? Don and I already have the best life ever. So, today as it happened, we massaged each other. Good for our health, good for the environment, and costs nothing!

To let politicians "solve" our problems is always going to fail because their agenda is always going to be power or money—or both.

Ha. I am an anarchist. I even think it might work, as everybody does want to be happy and from Burning Man, I learned that there is always going to be the rotten apple. Well, let's collectively look after that one . . .

I will smile and wave to my wayward neighbour—little acts of kindness to the people who least deserve it.

Something like that

I would love to hear your view.

Jozien xox

My name is Jozien. I am a wildflower buff, a connoisseur of mountain tops, and always a student.

I live with my husband in the woods in Yukon, Canada

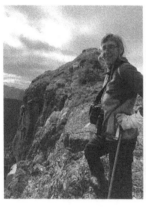 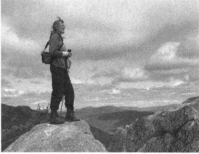

*   *   *

Hi Belle:

During COVID, I decided to go to a park in North Vancouver called "Kings Mill Walk Park. I called it Harbourside Park.

I bring my chair, my music stand, and my ukulele. I started by myself, and the next thing you know, my sister, Maureen joined me, and then a few others joined me.

We go and play and sing in the park EVERY single day at 2:30 p.m., winter, summer, spring, and fall. When it's raining, we go to the North Shore Library where there's a covered shelter.

It's been a Godsend . . . people come by and sing with us, some musicians, some simply soulful. It has saved my life. I don't ever think about my cancer or my blindness. I do have a hard time reading the music notes now, but who cares if I'm not playing the right notes?

It is soooooo much fun meeting more and more people as they are walking by. Some like to stop and sing along with us.

COVID really hasn't affected me too much, I'm having the time of my life just playing and singing.

God Bless,
Carol MacDowall
Carol and friends

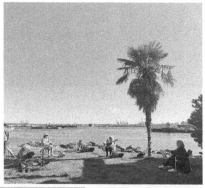

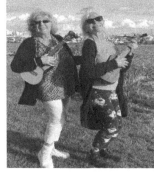
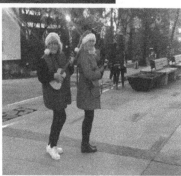

*   *   *

FAITH FAMILY AND FRIENDS
HOW THE VIRUS STOLE CHRISTMAS
By Stephanie Sackett-Converse
Sent By Spencer Piller

'Twas late in '19 when the virus began
Bringing chaos and fear to all people,
Each land they were sick, hospitals full,
Doctors o'rwhelmed, nobody in school.
As winter gave way to the promise of spring,
The virus raged on, touching peasant and king.
People hid in their homes from enemy unseen.

242

They You-Tubed and Zoomed, social-distanced, and cleaned.
April approached and churches were closed,
"There won't be an Easter," the world supposed.
"There won't be church services, and egg hunts are out.
No reason for new dresses when we can't go about."
Holy Week started, as bleak as the rest.
The world was focused on masks and on tests.
"Easter can't happen this year," it proclaimed.
"Online and at home, it just won't be the same."
Monday, Thursday, Good Friday, the days came and went.
The virus pressed on; it just would not relent.
The world woke Sunday and nothing had changed.
The virus still menaced, the people, estranged.
"Pooh pooh to the saints," the world was grumbling.
"They're finding out now that no Easter is coming.
"They're just waking up! We know just what they'll do!
Their mouths will hang open a minute to two,
And then all the saints will all cry boo-hoo.
"That noise," said the world, "will be something to hear."
So it paused and the world put a hand to its ear.
And it did hear a sound coming through all the skies.
It started down low, then it started to rise.
But the sound wasn't depressed.
Why, this sound was triumphant!
It couldn't be so!
But it grew with abundance!
The world started around, popping its eyes.
Then it shook! What it saw was a shocking surprise!
Every saint in every nation, the tall and the small,

Was celebrating Jesus in spite of it all!

It hadn't stopped Easter from coming! It came!

Somehow or other, it came just the same!

And the world with its life quite stuck in quarantine.

Stood puzzling and puzzling.

"Just how can it be?"

"It came without bonnets, it came without bunnies,

It came without egg hunts, cantatas or money."

Then the world thought of something it hadn't before.

"Maybe Easter," it thought, "doesn't come from a store.

Maybe Easter, perhaps, means a little bit more."

And what happened then?

Well . . . the story's not done.

What will YOU do?

Will you share that one

Or two or more people needing hope in this night?

Will you share the source of your life in this fight?

The churches are empty – but so is the tomb,

And Jesus is victor over death, doom, and gloom.

So this year at Easter, let this be our prayer,

As the virus still rages all around, everywhere.

May the world see hope when it looks at God's people.

May the world see the church is not a building or steeple.

May the world find Faith in Jesus's death and resurrection,

May the world find Joy in a time of dejection.

May 2020 be known as the year of survival,

But not only that . . .

Let it start a revival.

*   *   *

You Know You've Been Isolating Too Long If . . .
By Neil Holland
(JUST A LITTLE BIT OF HUMOUR)

Just be careful because people are going crazy from being in lockdown! Actually, I've just been talking about this with the microwave and toaster while drinking coffee, and we all agreed that things are getting bad. I didn't mention anything to the washing machine, as she puts a different spin on everything. Certainly not the fridge as he is acting cold and distant. In the end, the iron straightened me out as she said everything will be fine; no situation is too pressing. The vacuum was very unsympathetic . . . told me to just suck it up, but the fan was optimistic and hoped it would all soon blow over! The toilet looked a bit flushed when I asked its opinion and didn't say anything but the doorknob told me to get a grip. The front door said I was unhinged and so the curtains told me to . . . yes, you guessed it: pull myself together"

* * *

A Happy Place
By Neall Ryon

Find me a place where Mother Earth lives.
For I will be happy there.

Find me a place where the pine trees whisper their song,
and I will be happy there.

Find me a place where winter means snow and cold, crisp clear nights, and I will be happy there.

Find me a place where stillness exists, where gentle breezes blow.
Find me a place where fire-weed blossoms in the spring,
a place where cities don't exist and cool streams still flow
And I will be happy there.

Find me a place where nature is alive and well,
and bury me in that place,
for I will be happy there.

*　　*　　*

DOGS ARE AMAZING
Belle Curd

Regina, my helper, has a dog and a cat. I like pets but these two absolutely ignore me. I knew the dog was amazing as Regina took him down to the beach everyday, winters, summers and he goes in for a swim. Regina dries him off with a towel and thus goes his routine. He is 14 years old and apparently, he likes to be rubbed by the fellow walkers along the sand. However me no, not until last night. Coming home last night we all met at the front entrance.

He came up to me and allowed me to scratch his back with vigor for the first time. Regina was surprised. Then he decided to get to know me as dogs sometimes do and he sniffed where dogs sniff each other. Regina called him away but he came back. It was as if he were trying to protect me and tell me something. It was uncanny.

Regina's cat, Sparkles, has also been shy. The other night Regina gave me a small nibbler to feed her. She (the cat) wouldn't take the treat from my palm but nibbled it hungrily from the tips of my fingers. Then last night I had the door ajar ever so little and Sparkles made her way in and came up rather close to me to get her treat. I didn't have one so she took off but I'll just have to get her one for next time. Animals are so intelligent. She had come down right on cue, right on time. Searching for her treat.

You hear of animals mainly dogs acting in such a way as to trigger finding of diseases in people such as cancer. It made one shutter to think of it as I do have problems bleeding and sores not healing. Otherwise, I am in fairly good shape for my age and prior operations.

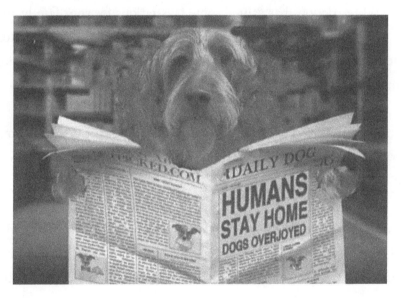

Dog Wisdom

Much thanks to all those who helped us with the Covid 19 Echoes book. We couldn't have done it without you. We had a lot of difficulty picking a title for the book, but it has come out very well. Some suggested Echoes and others suggested the Pandemic and Me. We hope no one has been affected during this stressful period. A portion of the profits from this book will go to charity. Thank you.

Special appreciation:

Marlene York. Our deepest sympathies go out to my niece Marlene and her husband and family for their loss, and they took the time to let me know. Thank you for contributing to the book.

Yvonne Gibbon. Thanks for giving us your covid experience. Sorry that COVID restrictions has caused some frustrations for your family and not being able to go to your granddaughters wedding in Washington state. I hope by now you have been able to visit the newly married couple.

Hetty Willeumier. Thank you, my good friend, for the depths of your story. You have helped us greatly. You are a great influence on all those around you.

Cynthia Sharpe. Thank you for your "Alone and Together" story and your "Even if These Are Our Last Days" poetry. They were very insightful to read. Your picture in British Columbia in spite of the pandemic was a delight to read.

Cynthia Hadden. We loved your thoughts on Covid and the quote "permeates our thoughts, our actions. Confusing us all" certainly express we have had over the past year and more. Keep up your interests over there in the sunshine coast of British Columbia.

Del Lobo. Thank you for your one act play. That was special. You are very talented. Keep up the good work British Columbia. It is amazing how those around us can be such an example to those who need a lift up.

Laurel Sukkau. Thank you for helping us find ways of feeling good in spite of this pandemic around us. Your smiling face will always brighten the world around you.

Jozien. Thank you Jozien, we appreciate your story all the way from Yukon in Northern Canada. Good health to you and good health to the planet too.

Mike Sackett. Thank you, Mike. Glad to have you aboard. Add this to the many enterprises you have accomplished. You will happy to learn that a portion of the proceeds from this co-operative effort we ordinary lovers of writing and our love of mankind have accomplished, will go to charity.

Carol and Donald Mcdowall and friends. Your cheery writeup was gladly received. All that read it will be made happier in spite of Covid. We will welcome the summer when we can be more out in the sunshine and not cooped inside.

Spencer Piller. Thank you for the receipt of your photos and verses by Stephanie Converse. I was not able to get her personal permission to use it but I assume it was taken from an email and that she would want the whole world to read it and enjoy it under her name.

Neil Holland. I'm assuming your comical piece came in through my son, and your long-time friend, Douglas Hogg. Our readers may need all the humor these days that they can get. Very clever. Glad to share.

Unknown. GLOBAL HEALTH. Thank you to whoever wrote this piece. I'd like to say it was me but on closer scrutiny I cannot claim it but it is a great. Whoever you are please receive our congratulations.

Neall Ryon. "A HAPPY PLACE." That was a lovely poem. Thank you so much. Like all our contributors, you have a special talent.

Maxwell. Thank you for the wonderful comment. "Belle, COVID 19 ECHOES is such an inspiring accomplishment—full of multi-generational insight, optimism, and compassion. I'm honored to be your editor, and do let me know if you have any questions whatsoever. Stay safe, and keep enjoying the bananas! All the best and more, Maxwell"

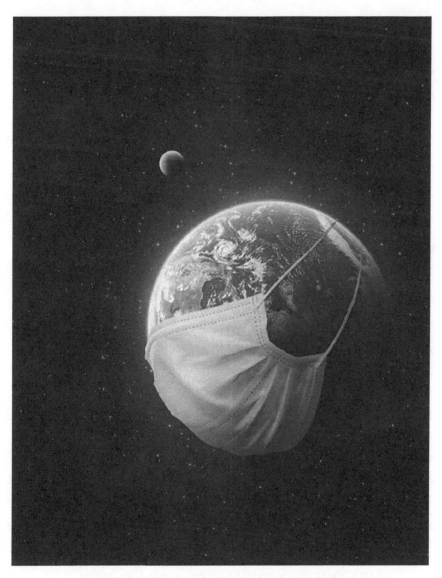

THE WORLD WITH A FACE MASK ON

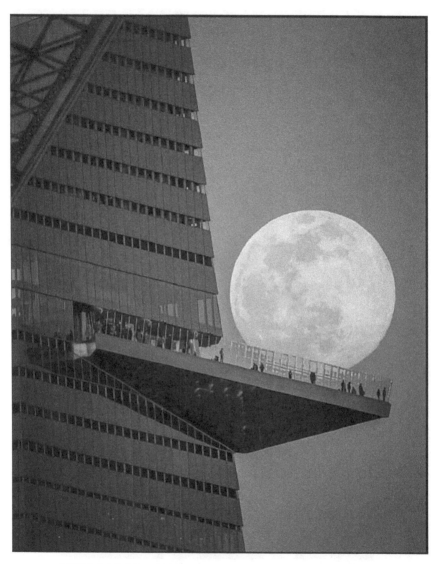

FULL MOON AT THE SIDE OF A TALL BUILDING

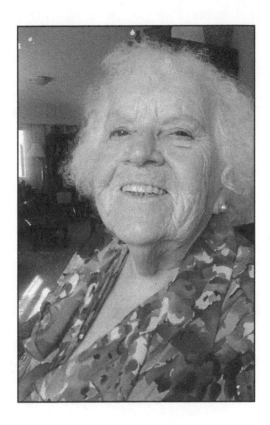

AUTHOR, BELLE MAYNARD CURD

Belle Maynard Curd was born in 1929 who now lives in Vancouver, British Columbia, mother of three, formally wife of Radar Rate William Hogg in the Royal Canadian Navy, widowed and remarried to Charles Curd also a sailor in the British Navy, a bricklayer in life. She is the grandmother of ten and the great grandmother of five.

Belle is known for her good humour at work. She loves writing, and she will never run out of books to write before she runs out of years to live. She is thankful for every blessing that has been bestowed upon her. Her aims in life are to keep on writing, learning and helping others.

CPSIA information can be obtained
at www.ICGtesting.com
Printed in the USA
BVHW072233050123
655436BV00001B/1

9 781685 366070